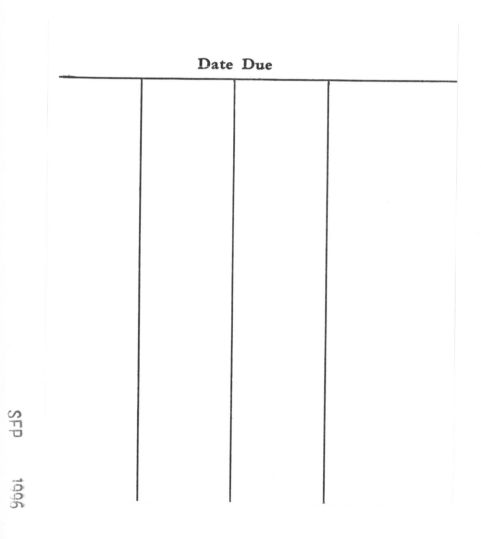

Law and the Team Physician

Elizabeth M. Gallup, MD, JD

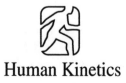

Human Kinetics

Library of Congress Cataloging-in-Publication Data

Gallup, Elizabeth M.
    Law and the team physician / Elizabeth M. Gallup.
       p.   cm.
    Includes index.
    ISBN 0-87322-662-3
    1. Sports medicine--Law and legislation--United States.
  I. Title.
  KF2910.S65G35   1995
  344.73'0412--dc20
  [347.304412]   93-47607
                                     CIP

ISBN: 0-87322-662-3

Acquisitions Editor: Rick Frey, PhD; **Developmental Editors:** Ann Brodsky, Mary E. Fowler; **Assistant Editors:** John Wentworth, Anna Curry, Hank Woolsey, Kezia E. Endsley; **Copyeditor:** Ginger Rodriguez; **Proofreader:** Sue Fetters; **Indexer:** Theresa J. Schafer; **Production Director:** Ernie Noa; **Typesetter:** Ruby Zimmerman; **Text Designer:** Jody Boles; **Layout Artist:** Denise Lowry; **Cover Designer:** Jack Davis; **Printer:** Braun-Brumfield

This book is intended to be a legal guide for the team physician. It is in no way intended nor should it be taken as legal advice. Before using any sample documents or pursuing a specific legal course, advice should be sought from legal counsel.

Printed in the United States of America   10 9 8 7 6 5 4 3 2 1

Human Kinetics
P.O. Box 5076, Champaign, IL 61825-5076
1-800-747-4457

Canada: Human Kinetics, Box 24040, Windsor, ON N8Y 4Y9
1-800-465-7301 (in Canada only)

Europe: Human Kinetics, P.O. Box IW14, Leeds LS16 6TR, England
(44) 532 781708

Australia: Human Kinetics, 2 Ingrid Street, Clapham 5062, South Australia
(08) 371 3755

New Zealand: Human Kinetics, P.O. Box 105-231, Auckland 1
(09) 309 2259

This book is dedicated to my mother, Juanita Gallup Penney, and my stepfather, Milton Herbert Penney.

Contents

Preface

Sports medicine is a discrete entity in the practice of medicine. The special legal duties and the liabilities team physicians have—whether they are primary care practitioners or specialists, volunteers, or professionals—are rapidly developing areas of law. This development occurs on the heels of a recent increase in the frequency and severity of lawsuits filed against physicians in general. *Law and the Team Physician* examines the areas of liability team physicians may face in their delivery of care. It also is a useful reference for educational administrators and lawyers who work with schools and colleges.

Sports-related litigation is on the rise in this country, involving not only professional athletes but also amateur athletes. *Law and the Team Physician* discusses by chapter the various areas of legal concern to team physicians. At the end of each chapter a section on practical considerations recapitulates the information, distilling it into easy application for the team physician's practice.

The first chapter deals with the concept, duties, and responsibilities of a team physician, discussing the standard of care by which a court of law might measure team physicians. It gives guidelines and parameters for team physicians and cites their possible effects. Chapter 2 discusses the anatomy of a lawsuit and the legal theory of negligence. The third chapter identifies the "Good Samaritan," a protective concept aimed at limiting a team physician's liability, and embraced by state legislatures to recruit physicians to the athletic sidelines.

We next consider the related concepts of contributory negligence, informed consent, assumption of risk, exculpatory waivers, and comparative negligence. Each of these legal doctrines can affect a team physician's ultimate liability. Chapter 5 examines the duties and liabilities team physicians encounter in the preparticipation examination, including the legal implications emanating from the decision to deny an athlete clearance. We then turn, in chapter 6, to the difficult decisions about when an athlete should be allowed to return to play.

Legal aspects of the choice, maintenance, application, and prescription of protective equipment comprise chapter 7, along with reviewing the suggested contents of the team physician's bag. Chapter 8 identifies common catastrophic injuries and conditions and considers their legal aspects in sports medicine. Drug use in sports is widespread, as chapter 9 shows through statistics, giving rise to the role team physicians may have in identifying, counseling, and testing athletes who use drugs.

Magic Johnson has brought HIV to the forefront of athletics. In chapter 10 we look at identifying, treating, and maintaining confidentiality of the HIV-positive athlete and the legal ramifications of these decisions. Chapter 11 considers the unique legal relationships that professional and collegiate team physicians encounter because of their paid employment by a college, university, or professional team. Finally, chapter 12 addresses specific risk management techniques team physicians may employ to minimize the possibilities of lawsuits.

The goal of this book is to provide team physicians with an overview of applicable law. It is also designed to encourage team physicians to continue to provide a valuable service to society, even in the face of a potential lawsuit.

Acknowledgments

Special thanks to Cyd Slayton, Walter Ricci, M.D., Tripti Kataria, M.D., Adam Skinner, M.D., Lisa Miller, and Linda Harrington.

Introduction

This book is designed to be a legal *guide* for those who act as team physicians for junior high, high school, collegiate, or professional sports teams. Note the word *guide*—team physicians can use the information they find here to guide them through the legal morass that faces all practitioners of medicine. The book is a guide to the legal principles that have an impact on some of the unique problems a team physician faces.

Law is quite different from medicine in some very important respects. Often in medicine, answers are clear-cut, diagnoses are straightforward, and treatment plans are clear and well-defined. In law, often the reverse is true. Law almost always demands that the benefits and detriments of each option and alternative be balanced. Law involves looking at any given situation from all possible angles; in medicine the tactic is often to zero in on the most likely possibility.

To determine the legally appropriate course involves reviewing legal precedent—case law—and applying it to the current situation. But no two cases are exactly alike, just as no two given clinical situations are exactly alike. Another problem is a dearth of case law in sports medicine. From 1970 to 1985 25 lawsuits were filed on behalf of athlete-plaintiffs who sustained head or neck injuries playing football. Eleven of these lawsuits were decided for the plaintiffs, awarding a total of $45.8 million. However, most of the suits were paid by helmet manufacturers—in only a few isolated instances have school districts, coaches, athletic associations, and physicians been successfully sued.[1] Twenty-five lawsuits in 15 years is a very small number compared with the number of athletes who participate in sports at all levels. Thus there are not many cases from which to elicit case law applicable to the duties of team physicians, and this book generally represents the extrapolation of case law. In other words, it takes information derived from some lawsuits not directly on point and uses this information to develop suggested guidelines for the team physician to follow.

Although lawsuits against team physicians are rare they are increasing in number. With the litigious nature of society, physicians who volunteer or who are paid to be team physicians are potentially vulnerable to legal action in several areas. Most sports medicine litigation involves the initial management of catastrophic injuries or decisions about when an athlete can return to sports participation.[1] Having guidelines in place and communicating well with the team, the athletes, athletic trainers, coaches, and parents are important in decreasing the potential for being sued.

As in medicine, in law there are no guarantees—following all the guidelines in this book will not guarantee that you will not be sued. People sue doctors all the time; frivolous lawsuits are on the rise. However, following the guidelines in this book may decrease the likelihood that you will be sued and make it less likely that you'll be found liable if you are sued.

The legal aspects of sports medicine is an evolving area. As a physician and a lawyer, I have functioned as a team physician at both the high school and collegiate levels and as an attorney who has counseled physicians. I hope to use my experience to give you a new perspective on how the law may affect the practice of sports medicine. I also hope to illustrate the concept that practicing sports medicine to minimize legal risks is also the best way to serve the athletes who are our patients.

This book is also focused on the needs of the high school team physician although many of the principles also apply to collegiate and professional team physicians, and I discuss issues pertinent specifically to them in a separate chapter. I chose this focus because of the predominance of team physicians who devote their time to caring for various high school athletic teams. The issues faced by volunteer high school team physicians can sometimes be a world apart, legally, from those faced by college and professional team physicians. High school team physicians typically serve on a volunteer basis, are not employees of the school system, are identifiable and active members of the general community, and have developed ongoing physician-patient relationships with many members of the community. This is quite distinct from the relationships that occur when the team physician is on the payroll. The care and sacrifice of these high school volunteer team physicians promote healthy athletic participation for millions of athletes every year.

---

[1](1992). Team physicians are vulnerable to legal action in several areas. *Family Practice News,* **22,** 7.

CHAPTER 1

The Team Physician: Definition, Role, and Training

During a Saturday night basketball game, a first-string forward makes a cutting move at the top of the key to avoid a block by the defensive guard and immediately goes down with an ankle sprain. He is removed to the sidelines where his leg is elevated, iced, and ace-wrapped by the team physician, a general practitioner whose son is also on the team. The athlete is placed on crutches and advised not to bear weight for 3 days. The athlete does not use his crutches because he thinks they make him look weak. Instead he hobbles around on the ankle until the team physician examines him the following Wednesday. The ankle is edematous and discolored. The team physician advises the athlete that he cannot participate in Friday night's game. The athlete protests, and the coach pressures the team physician to let the athlete play: Without him the team will surely lose to their arch rivals.

Finally the team physician relents, allowing the team's most valuable player to participate, telling the athlete, however, to be sure to wear high tops to give extra support to the ankle. The athlete plays Friday night wearing his regular low tops because the high tops hurt. After twisting his ankle on the first play, the athlete is carried out and the town's orthopedic surgeon diagnoses a grade III ankle sprain requiring surgery to stabilize.

Questions:

▮ To what standard is the team physician held—a general practitioner, a team physician with specialized training in sports medicine, an orthopedic surgeon, or a primary care physician who has a certificate of added qualification?

- If the team physician is sued, what kind of physician can testify against him—an orthopedic surgeon, another general practitioner, a family physician, or a Certificate of Added Qualification (CAQ) primary care physician?
- Was it permissible to treat the star athlete differently than a third-stringer with a similar severe ankle sprain?
- Was it appropriate for the coach to pressure the team physician, and for the team physician to accede to the pressure?
- Is the team physician more liable because he did not follow the well-known guideline of adequately stabilizing the injured ankle before allowing the athlete to return to play?

The team physician concept is a broad one. It can include many different duties and responsibilities. Team physicians come from all different specialties, assume different relationships to the teams they serve, and have different responsibilities. To avoid questions of the team physician's responsibilities, a contract is extremely useful—it can spell out the parameters under which the team physician functions and can clearly denote the team physician's responsibilities to all parties involved. A contract helps define the role a team physician will play.

Who Are Team Physicians?

Sports medicine was once considered a passing fancy of physicians who dabbled in the field when they had children participating on a team. Sports medicine has now evolved into a more distinct area of medicine although it still is not a recognized subspecialty and is not precisely defined. Many sports medicine practitioners act as team physicians,[1] a role that has gradually evolved over the past decade as more physicians began to devote more of their time to the care of athletes.[2] The variations in arrangements reached with physicians to provide medical care for athletic participants are virtually limitless.[1]

Team physicians come from the ranks of primary care specialties such as family practice, pediatrics, and internal medicine. Orthopedic surgeons and other specialists also act as team physicians. A 1987 survey by *Physician and Sports Medicine* of 29,000 team physicians revealed that 23% were family physicians, 17% were orthopedists, 13% were general practitioners, and 4% were in the "other" category, which included osteopaths, internists, general surgeons, pediatricians, and obstetricians/gynecologists.

Usually, physicians become interested in sports medicine for one reason or another, and then seek out additional training in the area. For primary care physicians this extra training may be continuing medical education or a training fellowship which adds an additional 1 or 2 years to postdoctoral training. Orthopedic sports medicine fellowships are also available, and they also add 1 or 2 years of training.

A primary care physician or orthopedic surgeon is not required to complete a fellowship training to become a team physician. What is required to be a team physician is an interest and an effort to keep up to date and clinically competent in the area. Team physicians must also be willing and able to apply medical knowledge to athletics. Some team physicians, typically a primary care physician such as a family physician and an orthopedist,[3] share the duty of caring for a team.

The Certificate of Added Qualification in Sports Medicine

The American Board of Family Practice, the American Board of Internal Medicine, the American Board of Emergency Medicine, and the American Board of Pediatrics have developed an examination to certify candidates in sports medicine. The first examination for the certificate of added qualification in sports medicine was offered in 1993. To take the exam applicants must be certified by the appropriate specialty board and apply through a fellowship or a practice pathway.

To apply through a fellowship pathway, a candidate for the exam must have completed a minimum of 1 year in a sports medicine fellowship program associated with an accredited residency in family practice, internal medicine, pediatrics, or emergency medicine. The fellowships are accredited by the residency review committee of each specialty.

The practice pathway option will be available to candidates through 1999. After that, a 1-year sports medicine fellowship will be required for a candidate to be eligible for the examination. Practice eligibility consists of several elements, including 5 years of practice experience in which at least 20% of professional time is devoted to sports medicine. For purposes of the practice pathway, practice of sports medicine is defined as field supervision of athletes; emergency assessment and care of acutely injured athletes; diagnosis, treatment, management, and disposition of common sports injuries and illnesses; management of medical problems in the athlete; rehabilitation of ill and injured athletes; and prescribing exercise as treatment. In addition, candidates must have participated in 30 hours of the American Medical Association's Category I (or its equivalent) in sports medicine–related continuing medical education during the past five years.[4]

More and more team physicians will come from the ranks of physicians with the added certificate of qualifications. This may have an effect on the legal standard against which the physician will be measured if he is sued, a topic that will be discussed in more detail later in this chapter.

Traveling Team Physicians and Licensure

Team physicians may travel with athletic teams to competition sites away from home, which may take them out of the state in which they are licensed to practice medicine. In general, state laws allow physicians licensed in other states to practice medicine occasionally as long as the physician does not maintain an office or hold out as a licensed practitioner in that state.[5] However, team physicians are not permitted to admit athletes to hospitals, in part because of being unlicensed but also because the team physician would not have hospital privileges in a state where he is not licensed. For maximum protection, you should ascertain what the state laws are regarding the occasional practice of medicine by unlicensed physicians in states where you will be traveling.

The Team Physician's Role

Team physicians have a unique role in the athletic medicine setting.[6] They may be friends and advisors to the athletes, role models, and part of the group of school personnel that selects equipment. The school, community, parents, coaches, and team expect them to make major decisions about athletes' health, qualifications to join the team, and ability to participate safely. They may have to decide whether an athlete can participate from the office, at the practice field, or at the game. Many of these decisions are made under the intense pressure of a game situation and involve a critical time factor. Ramifications of the team physician's decisions are not only immediate, such as keeping an individual athlete out of a game, but also long-term, affecting the outcome of a game, the team's standing in a league, and the athletes' and coaches' future careers.[6]

The Team Physician's Duty and Standard of Care

The team physician's duty is to take care of the individual athletes on the team and the team as a whole. The physician best suited to be a team physician is one who understands the physical and emotional needs of the athlete in the context of the sport and who maintains broad, up-to-date knowledge of the musculoskeletal system, growth and development, the cardiorespiratory system, gynecology, dermatology, neurology, pharmacology, and exercise science.

Recognize Sports-Specific Injuries and Regulations

The competent team physician will generally be familiar with common injuries that occur in the sport in which the team participates. Some of the common sports-specific injuries are noted in Table 1.1.

Table 1.1   Sports-Specific Injuries

Sport	Common injury types	Most common sites	Special comments
Soccer	Strains, sprains, contusions, dislocations, and fractures	Lower extremities	Most injuries are the result of physical contact between players
Football	Sprains, dislocations, strains, head injury, c-spine injuries	Hand, knee, ankle	High incidence of c-spine and head injuries relative to other sports
Rugby	Sprains, dislocations, strains, head injury, c-spine injuries	Head and neck, upper limbs	High incidence of c-spine and head injuries relative to other sports
Basketball	Sprains, strains, stress injuries	Ankles, knees	
Volleyball	Sprains, strains, stress injuries	Ankles, fingers, knees, shoulders	Suprascapular neuropathy may also be seen; injuries most often occur during blocking and diving for a ball
Baseball	Dislocations, tendinitis, sprains, strains	Fingers, shoulders, elbows, ankles, knees	Most injuries occur to pitchers and catchers or while diving for a ball or sliding to a base
Ice hockey	Contusions, lacerations, fractures, dislocations	Face, dental	Injuries frequently caused by contact with puck, stick, or skate
Racket sports	Strains, muscle rupture, overuse injuries	Lower extremities, achilles tendon	
Track and field	Strains, sprains, overuse injuries	Knee, ankle, lower back, shoulder	Varied because wide variety of sports involved
Gymnastics	Sprains, fractures	Upper and lower extremities, back	Many injuries involve bar and balance beam

Note. From Kujala, U., Heinonen, O., Lehto, M., et al. (1988). Equipment, drugs, and problems of the team physician. *Sports Medicine,* **6,** 197-209.

The team physicians must also keep apprised of sports-specific regulations. Many sports have special rules for medical tasks before competition, such as specialized taping regulations in boxing and certain track and field events and use of orthoses in contact sports, and regulations regarding on-field examination of athletes. Team physicians must also understand regulations governing the use of drugs in competitive sports.[7]

Have an Organizational Plan

Another duty is to have an organizational plan for a team approach to the injured athlete. The organizational plan should include

1. identification of appropriately trained personnel to assist in the provision of on-site emergency medical care,
2. provision of adequate on-site emergency equipment,
3. determination of adequate emergency transportation with appropriately trained personnel on-site or available on call,
4. development of appropriate communication mechanisms to summon emergency transportation,
5. identification of appropriate hospital facilities with well-trained personnel, and
6. identification of appropriate consultative services.[8]

See Appendix A for a more detailed checklist for the team physician.

Keep Adequate Records

As in all areas of medicine, there is no substitute for adequate record keeping. Proper documentation is a component of competent medical care. Without it physicians face the possibility, if not the probability, of losing a lawsuit in which they know they were not negligent. Documentation is more thoroughly addressed in chapter 12, which deals with risk management.

Confidentiality and Allegiance

Another important duty is confidentiality and allegiance. The general public is often very interested in athletes, their physical abilities, and their injuries, and the press and other interested individuals may ask the team physician for this information. However, the team physician must remember that her allegiance first and foremost is to the athlete. The American Medical Association states that the interest of the patient, here the athlete, is paramount in the practice of medicine.[9] These principles of medical ethics admonish physicians not to reveal confidence entrusted to them unless required to do so by law or to protect the welfare of the individual or the community.[18] Therefore, the team physician should not reveal any information about an athlete unless the law requires her to do so, which may occur if the athlete later sues a team physician, or unless an athlete gives the team physician permission to reveal information. If a team physician does give information about an athlete's condition to someone, he may be subject to liability for defamation, invasion of privacy, breach of a confidential relationship, or the like. Hence, the physician should be extremely careful about what information she gives and to whom she gives it.

Practice in a Competent Manner

Team physicians have a duty to practice medicine in a competent manner, as measured against a standard of care. The general standard of care, applicable to all physicians, is that the physician must exercise that degree of care, skill, and diligence ordinarily exercised by other physicians under the same or similar circumstances.[10] Applied to the conduct of a team physician, the issue is what the standard of care is for a team physician. This issue revolves around the question of what the generally accepted duties of team physicians are.

First and foremost, the team physician is responsible for the medical supervision of athletes, which includes the following duties among others: managing athletic injuries, performing participation examinations, making recommendations regarding participation in sports and treatment or rehabilitation, and advising about conditioning and the use of protective equipment.

Though less common, team physicians may also be responsible for administrative functions such as developing guidelines for coaches and athletic trainers (e.g., guidelines regarding precautions for exercise in a high heat, high humidity environment); supervising the school's athletic trainers; arranging for emergency equipment; evaluating and recommending protective equipment and advising on how to use it correctly; and educating coaches, athletic trainers, injured athletes, and parents.[3]

The most frequent allegation against physicians is failure to diagnose.[11] Although failure to diagnose is a serious allegation for any physician, it can have far-reaching ramifications for the team physician. If the team physician misdiagnoses a condition as more serious than it actually is and, as a result, the player's career suffers, then the team physician may be liable to the athlete. In addition, liability could also arise if the team physician misdiagnoses a condition as less serious than it is, and consequently the athlete exacerbates the problem, harming his or her career. This liability can possibly include future economic losses, which may include loss of a scholarship and loss of future earnings that could have been received if the athlete had gone on to a professional career.[12] Failure to diagnose in preparticipation examinations is more fully discussed in chapter 5.

The general concept of the team physician's duties and responsibilities and its relation to the standard of care is constantly evolving. The standard of care is used in a court of law in the event that a team physician is sued. Without a universally accepted definition of what a team physician is, what the role of the team physician is, or what the standard of care is, the standard of care is ultimately determined in the courtroom based on the testimony of experts.[13] If a team physician is sued and the lawsuit makes it to trial, he will have an expert testify on his behalf as to what the standard of care is in the same or similar circumstances as in the incident that gave rise to the lawsuit. An expert will also testify on behalf of the plaintiff, the athlete who was treated by the team physician, or her family. This expert may claim that a different standard of care should have been practiced in the same or similar circumstances. It is from the two competing standards testified to in court that the jury ultimately determines whether or not the team physician was negligent in the incident giving rise to the lawsuit.

Team physicians should be extremely careful to avoid misleading the team, parents, and school about their capabilities—they should make their limitations known in advance.[14] It is also essential to let the team, coaches, and parents know to what extent the team physician will care for athletes. Physicians in general are free to limit their working hours, radius of travel, locations at which services are rendered, and scope of services, just as they are free to set priorities among patients' needs.[1] Likewise, team physicians should be entitled to limit the occasions during which they will render services. A team physician for a high school football team may agree to attend the games and to treat medical conditions that arise during the game. He may, however, decline to treat injuries or conditions that arise during practice or to provide general medical care to the athletes unrelated to injuries that occur due to their athletic participation.[1] It is essential to let the team, the coaches, and the parents know these limitations at the beginning of the season, when such limitations would not otherwise reasonably be apparent to a similarly situated patient.[15]

Even though team physicians can limit the scope of their undertaking and thus the duty of care they are responsible for providing, they cannot do so to any extent they choose. If the team physician has a physician-patient relationship with an athlete because of an injury or other incident, she cannot limit her responsibilities to that athlete when to do so would unreasonably endanger the athlete's health.

Are Team Physicians Specialists In the Eyes of the Law?

Another question to be addressed is whether team physicians should be deemed specialists for purposes of the standard of care required. This issue comes into play in determining what experts can testify on behalf of and against a team physician who is a defendant in a lawsuit. At this point it is not possible to automatically categorize all team physicians as de facto specialists with a sports medicine "specialty." Neither sports medicine nor the team physician role has been designated a discreet specialty or subspecialty by the Council on Medical Education of the American Medical Association (AMA).[16] The actual training and level of involvement of physicians serving as team physicians vary widely, as previously discussed. Team physicians may be orthopedic specialists, primary care physicians, or physicians in any other specialty.[17] The picture is further complicated by the development of the certificate of added qualification in sports medicine and by the formation of new medical societies specifically addressing the needs of primary care physicians who serve as team physicians and of orthopedic surgeons who take on that role.

If a physician holds himself out as a "specialist" in sports medicine, then it may be that he will be held to a higher standard of care in the courtroom. In other words, if a team physician holds herself out as a specialist, the court may hold her to the standard of care that would have been practiced by a physician who had earned the certificate of added qualification in sports medicine (a specialist in the field) regardless of whether or not the physician in question had received the certificate of added qualification.

Some states require experts who testify in court either on behalf of or against the defendant physician to be in the same specialty as the defendant physician. If this is applied to a team physician who has called himself a "specialist" in the field of sports medicine, then the expert testifying for him will, in the future, have a certificate of added qualification whether or not the defendant team physician does.

The Evolution of Practice Parameters and Guidelines

The 1980s may well be known as the decade of the standard of care.[18] The trend of developing standards, also called guidelines or practice parameters, will certainly continue. Many medical organizations, the federal government, states, managed-care entities, and physician groups are developing standards by which to practice for a variety of reasons, including containing costs, insuring quality, and lowering professional liability exposure.[19]

In 1986 very specific standards of practice for monitoring surgical patients during anesthesia were developed at Harvard Medical School. The developers of the anesthesia standards noted that such efforts could

1. improve patient care while reducing the number of malpractice claims,
2. enhance the detection of relatively low-frequency events that are potentially hazardous to patients,
3. establish a means for objective evaluation of service provision, and
4. establish a precedent for ongoing standard efforts.[20]

Since these standards have been in place, malpractice insurance premiums for anesthesiologists have gradually decreased.[20]

Practice standards or guidelines have also been developed in sports medicine. The American Academy of Pediatrics, AMA, and American College of Sports Medicine have all developed guidelines that may affect team physicians (the ACSM's have been published in *ACSM's Guidelines for Team Physicians*). Although it can be argued that guidelines are different than standards, in reality guidelines will be used in the courtroom as a measuring device in the same manner as standards are.

The legal effects of setting standards is generally beneficial to the medical profession rather than a significant threat of liability. As we discussed, defining relevant medical criteria from which to designate a standard of care involves a great deal of uncertainty—what type of specialist practices sports medicine, what limitations were known, and so on. Formally stated standards make designating a standard of care more certain. If specific standards of care have been established, they are more easily replicated in legal proceedings and may contribute to a consistent rule of liability.

To determine the appropriate standard of care against which a defendant team physician will be measured, courts utilize the testimony of expert witnesses, accrediting agencies' standards, statutes and official regulations, learned treatises (such as medical textbooks or articles), and, finally, policies and prescriptions from professional organizations and societies.[22] These policies and prescriptions from professional organizations and societies are another source of practice parameters or practice guidelines. The development of clinically based written standards to reduce the frequency and severity of medical malpractice loss appears to be gaining popularity among many specialty-specific organizations and professional liability insurers.[21] The probative value of these standards to juries is increasing because most courts tend to recognize national standards rather than the usual custom or practice of providers in a particular locality or community.[21]

However, although clinical practice guidelines, practice parameters, and standards can diminish team physicians' liability, they may increase it in their early stages of development, when physicians may be unaware of them, or before they are really tested. For example, suppose a practice parameter or standard suggests that team physicians should act in a certain way. Further suppose that a team physician is a member of a specialty organization that wrote and distributed the practice guideline. If she did not follow the practice guideline and an athlete has been injured, it is likely that the attorney for the athlete will attempt to persuade the jury that the team physician did not follow the guideline written by her own specialty group and therefore was negligent in the treatment and care of the athlete.

The American College of Sports Medicine has published guidelines stating that the team physician should be involved with choosing the protective equipment worn by athletes who participate in sports.[8] In general, team physicians don't participate in choosing and fitting protective equipment worn by all athletes, such as football players' helmets or shoulder pads. If an athlete is injured and the injury can be ascribed to ill-fitting protective equipment, then the team physician may be named in a lawsuit because of the duty outlined in the standard written by the American College of Sports Medicine to participate in choosing and fitting protective equipment.

It is impossible to mention all the practice parameters, guidelines, and standards that may potentially apply to athletic team physicians. In general, team physicians should be aware of the practice parameters developed by the American College of Sports Medicine, the AMA, and their own specialty organizations. By keeping current and practicing according to the guidelines, team physicians will markedly reduce their potential exposure to liability.

The Team Physician's Contract

Team physicians should execute a contract with the school or sport entity.[23] This contract should specifically identify the physician as the team physician and the individual ultimately responsible for making determinations regarding the athletes' participation and medical care. The contract should also specifically delineate the job description of the team physician, including services to be provided and the person to whom the team physician reports.[3] A letter of agreement that sets forth the team physician's duties and responsibilities, rather than a formal contract, is sufficient to create contractual obligations and protection. A sample letter can be found in Figure 1.1.

The following sets forth agreement between _____
and _____ School System regarding the performance by _____ of the duties as team physician.
_____ agrees to be team physician for
_____ (football team, baseball team, etc.).
For these services _____ will receive no monetary
remuneration. _____ is not considered an employee of _____ School System, and
_____ School System exercises no con-
trol over the independent medical judgment of _____.

As the team physician, _____ has the
ultimate responsibility and authority regarding an athlete's ability to participate. This includes initial clearance for the athlete to participate as well as
clearance for return to participation. Services provided by the team physician
will be the performance of preparticipation physical examinations on athletes
desiring to participate in interscholastic sports, the presence of the team
physician at athletic events, and other services commonly provided by team
physicians. The team physician will communicate directly with the coach and
the athletic director of the school.

Date: _____ 19 ____   Signed _____
                                                    Physician

                                 Signed _____
                                         School System Representative

Figure 1.1   A sample letter of agreement.

Whether or not the team physician receives remuneration for time spent
should be specifically stated in a separate clause from any that specifies
reimbursement for monies expended on behalf of caring for the team. In
general, team physicians are more protected from lawsuits if they provide
their services gratis and are only reimbursed for monies spent. Chapter 3,
on the Good Samaritan concept, will discuss payment in depth.

Each state has separate statutes regarding contracts. Team physicians
should seek legal advice either from their own lawyers or from the legal
counsel for the school or the sports entity who is responsible for drawing
up the contract. Whatever legal counsel is used, the team physician should
make sure that the attorney is familiar with the law of the state applicable
to the practice of medicine.

Not only can the contract legally protect the team physician, but also it is often helpful when the inevitable arises—a disagreement between the team physician's opinion regarding an athlete's participation and an "outside" physician's opinion. If the contract specifies that the team physician makes the ultimate determination, it is of great value in dealing with the coach, parents, and athlete. The contract can also be the basis for demanding that the athlete who disagrees with the team physician's opinion about participation execute an exculpatory waiver or a risk release. Waivers and releases are fully discussed in chapter 4, on exculpatory waivers and assumption of risk.

Practical Considerations

Team physicians come from many different walks of medicine. Their backgrounds are varied—they may be orthopedic surgeons, be neurosurgeons, or come from a primary care field such as family practice, pediatrics, or internal medicine. Team physicians may belong to a variety of specialty organizations—an organization for their own specialty or an organization made up of different specialties such as the American College of Sports Medicine or the American Medical Society for Sports Medicine.

Because team physicians come from a variety of backgrounds and specialties, they are not held to one defining standard of care. Team physicians may be held to a standard of care determined in a court of law from testimony of expert witnesses, the use of practice guidelines and practice parameters, and the use of learned treatises, such as medical textbooks and medical articles. Expert witnesses may be drawn from the physician's same specialty or a different specialty; the specialty to which they must belong varies from state to state.

In general, the team physician should attempt to keep up with guidelines developed by his specialty society, the American Medical Association, the American College of Sports Medicine, and other sports-specific medical organizations. Commonly, if a team physician is a member of these organizations, then she is presumed to know and follow the organization's written guidelines.

No laundry list defines the duties of team physicians; they vary with the situation, the interest of the school system, and the team physician. But it is generally accepted that the team physician will have knowledge of the sport, of diagnosis and treatment of the more common sport-specific injuries, and of the special areas of the preparticipation exam required by the sport.

It is also generally accepted that the team physician will be available at the game, especially in sports where there is a high incidence of injury such as football, hockey, and soccer. Usually, it is the responsibility of the team physician to ascertain whether or not emergency personnel or an ambulance crew is available at the game and, if not, how to procure the dispatch of one.

The competent team physician will know when her scope of practice has been exceeded and when to refer accordingly. The team physician is generally expected to know the appropriate applications of protective equipment and proper conditioning and rehabilitation exercises.

The team physician should be extremely careful about divulging information about athletes under his care. The team physician has a physician-patient relationship with athletes and owes them the duty of confidentiality.

It is very important to execute a contract that specifically defines the scope of the team physician's responsibilities and remuneration. A contract can generally be prepared without much problem or expense—any expense is usually borne by the school or sports entity.

The most important responsibility after care of the athletes themselves is the responsibility of proper documentation. There is no substitute for documentation—and there is no escape from it either.

References

1. King, J.H. (1982, May). The duty and the standard of care for team physicians. *Houston Law Review*, **18**(4), 657-705, 681.
2. Gallup, E.M. (1991, November). Staying inbounds and out of court. *The Physician and Sports Medicine*, **19**(11), 145-148.
3. Mellion, M., Walsh, W., & Shelton, G. (1990). *The team physicians handbook* (pp. 1-6). St. Louis: Hanley and Belfus Inc. Mosby-Yearbooks.
4. American Board of Family Practice. (1992). Brochure describing the Certificates of Added Qualification in Sports Medicine. Lexington, KY: Author.
5. Herbert, D.L. (1991, October). Questions for the editors. *Sports Medicine Standard and Malpractice Reporter*, **3**(4), 73-74.
6. Pitt, M.B. (1987). Malpractice on the sidelines: Developing a standard of care for team sports physicians. *Journal of Communications and Entertainment Law*, **2**(3), 579-600.
7. Kujala, U.M., Heinonen, O.J., Lehto, M., Jarvinen, M., & Bergfeld, J.A. (1988). Equipment, drugs, and problems of the competition and team physician. *Sports Medicine*, **6**, 197-209.
8. Cantu, R., & Micheli, L. (1991). *American College of Sports Medicine's guidelines for the team physician* (pp. 97, 223-227). Philadelphia: Lea & Febiger.

9. American Medical Association Council on Ethical Affairs. (1989). *Current opinions of the Council on Ethical and Judicial Affairs* (p. 56). Chicago: American Medical Association.
10. Prosser, W. (1971). *The law of torts* (4th ed.) (pp. 161-164). St. Paul: West.
11. American Academy of Family Physicians Committee on Professional Liability. (1987). *Risk management and the family physician.* Kansas City, MO: American Academy of Family Physicians.
12. Prosser, W. (1971). *The law of torts* (4th ed.) (pp. 259-260). St. Paul: West.
13. American Medical Association. (1990). *Grand rounds on medical malpractice* (p. 58). Chicago: American Medical Association.
14. Sanbar, S.S., Pataki, L.J., Twardy, S., Thompson, C. (1989). Some medical legal aspects of sports medicine. *Legal Aspects of Medical Practice*, **6**(3), 5-9.
15. Hernandez v. Smith, 552 F.2d 142, 144-46 (5th Cir. 1977).
16. American Board of Medical Specialties Annual Report 6-7.
17. Hairsch, H. (1979, August). The generalist as team physician. *Physician and Sports Medicine*, **7**(1), 89.
18. American Medical Association. (1989, January 6). Year end review, medicine by the book. *AMA News*, 1-28.
19. Eichorn, J.G., et al. (1986). Standards for patient monitoring during anesthesia at Harvard Medical School. *JAMA*, **256**(8), 1017-1020.
20. Holzer, J.F. (1990, February). The advent of clinical standards for professional liability. *Quality Review Bulletin*, **16**(2), 71-79.
21. Weistart, J.C. (1985, December). Legal consequences of standards setting for competitive athletes with cardiovascular abnormalities. *Journal of the American College of Cardiology*, **6**(6), 1191-1197.
22. MacDonald, M.G., Meyer, K.C., & Sessig, B. (1988). *Health care law: A practical guide* (p. 329). New York: Matthew Bender.
23. Dyment, D. (1991). *Health care for young athletes* (2nd ed.) (pp. 172-187). Elk Grove, IL: American Academy of Pediatrics.

CHAPTER 2

The Anatomy of a Lawsuit and the Law of Negligence

(This chapter was written in conjunction with Brad Bradshaw, M.D., J.D.)

Dr. Jock, the local team physician, received a call from his friend at the courthouse saying that the sheriff was on his way to serve the doctor with notice that he was being sued by one of his former athlete-patients. Upon hearing this, Dr. Jock left his office and went to the hospital, ostensibly to see a patient but really to avoid the sheriff. The sheriff left the petition with Dr. Jock's nurse. Dr. Jock ignored the notice, never showed up for his lawsuit, and his athlete-turned-plaintiff won a judgment against him for $45,000.

Questions:

▮ What should Dr. Jock have done when he heard that the sheriff was on his way?

▮ What were the consequences of giving the petition to Dr. Jock's nurse and not to the doctor?

▮ When was the appropriate time for Dr. Jock to notify his medical malpractice insurance company of the lawsuit?

▮ Why was the doctor found liable for $45,000 in damages when he was never even present in the courtroom?

After a recent decline in the frequency and the severity of lawsuits against physicians in the United States, they are now increasing—in frequency and in the severity of damages awarded.[1] Team physicians are not immune to litigation; however, it is uncommon for a team physician, especially a high school or college team physician, to be sued for medical malpractice.

When physicians are sued, two thirds of the suits are dropped or settled without payment,[2] meaning that no settlement or award is made directly to the plaintiff who filed the lawsuit. Of the remaining lawsuits, only 5% go to court and result in verdicts against the practicing physician. Of these, only 1% ended in liability payments of $1 million or more. Therefore, team physicians are not often sued and, as for physicians practicing in all specialties, suits against them are not often successful.[2]

Medical Malpractice and the Law of Negligence

When team physicians are sued, the complaint typically is for practicing in a negligent fashion, that is, medical malpractice. For any physician to be successfully sued for medical malpractice, four key things must be proven. These four keys are the elements of negligence. Without proving each of the four elements, a plaintiff will not succeed in the medical malpractice suit against a physician. These four elements are

- duty,
- breach,
- causation, and
- damages.[3]

Duty

A successful suit must show team physicians to have a duty to practice competently when caring for an athlete. Usually the duty is apparent: The existence of a duty is the obvious fact that a physician has some responsibility to an athlete. There are rare cases, however, where duty is an issue. One such case involved a blind lady as patient. At the time of her appointment with the physician the would-be patient was told that her seeing-eye dog could not accompany her inside. The blind lady objected to leaving the dog outside, at which point she, her dog, and her child were refused admission. The initial trial decision was that the mere appointment with a physician does not establish a duty, but the Appeals Court said that whether a duty existed was up to the jury. In other words, the case would go to trial, and one of the issues the jury would decide was whether a duty even existed.[4] Generally, a duty is proven by showing that there was an established physician-patient relationship.[3]

The standard of care is an issue that involves what duty the team physician owes the athlete. The standard of care and how it is determined are discussed more fully in chapter 1. In general, however, the standard of care requires that the team physician possess and exercise the degree of skill and care ordinarily exercised by other health care professionals rendering the same type of medical service at issue in the particular case. For team physicians this means that a minimally competent team physician previously had done the same thing under the same or similar circumstances.[3]

Breach

The single most important issue in most medical malpractice cases, aside from the issue of adequate documentation, is the existence of a breach of duty.[5] In other words, if a duty, or a responsibility, was owed to the athlete, was there a violation of that responsibility? Simply put, a breach of the duty to the patient occurs where the care provided was substandard. An error in judgment itself is not malpractice if the error was a reasonable one. However, the judgment or data base used to formulate a clinical decision may be challenged as unreasonable or below an acceptable standard of care.[3] The court will determine the standard of care based on expert witness testimony.[5] The plaintiff's expert will testify what the standard should have been and that the standard was not met, resulting in a breach of the duty of care. The defendant's expert will testify that the standard was met and, thus, no breach occurred, explaining why it was met and on what basis the standard was determined. The jury is then left to decide between the two competing standards of care. Because the standards in sports medicine are fluid, as we discussed, many different guidelines can be brought into a case at this point.

Causation

The third of the four necessary elements to a malpractice action is causation. In malpractice actions, as well as in all negligence actions, there must be some reasonable connection between the negligent act and the damages the plaintiff suffered. In other words, the negligence must have caused the patient harm. Being negligent alone will not give rise to a malpractice action; the negligence must have caused the plaintiff harm.[6]

Suppose an athlete has a grade II ankle sprain and is returned to a football game without adequate taping or bracing to stabilize the ankle. This clearly is a negligent act by the team physician because team physicians of all specialties should know that grade II and grade III ankle sprains must be adequately stabilized by taping, bracing, or both, including the use of an air cast or air splint, before returning the athlete to the game. This is especially true if the athlete is involved in a sport that requires a lot of cutting, such as basketball and football. Now suppose the athlete, while going out for a pass, runs into the goal post, which causes concussion, a subdural hematoma, and death. The athlete's family may sue the physician for negligence. The court would examine the four elements of negligence. First, the physician had a duty to treat the athlete competently. The competent manner in which he should have treated the athlete was to stabilize the ankle with taping or an air splint. This was not done; therefore, the duty was breached. The damage in this case was the athlete's death. However, the athlete was killed by the subdural hematoma and not by the team physician's breach of duty to ensure that the ankle was stabilized. The lack of taping or adequately stabilizing the ankle did not cause the athlete to run into the goalpost and develop a subdural hematoma. Therefore, although the team physician's negligent action was a clear breach of duty, the breach had no causative effect on the damage, the death of the athlete. In a suit against the team physician for this negligent act, the plaintiff athlete's family should not be successful.

Damages

The final element of negligence is damages. This is the requirement that some actual harm must have been suffered by the patient. Negligence without damages will not result in a malpractice action.[7] The basic concept behind damages is that an injured person should be placed in the position he would have had if the injury had not occurred. U.S. courts have long recognized that the only damages available typically are money damages. Actual damages may be physical, financial, or emotional, but to award damages to injured plaintiffs, the court awards money.

Juries often differentiate between economic and noneconomic damages. Economic damages are those expenses that can readily be assigned an objective economic value, such as lost wages, medical bills, or the installation of wheelchair ramps. By contrast, noneconomic damages are attributable to the patient's emotional distress, physical pain and suffering, lack of consortium, or other largely subjective losses. Economic damages are measurable whereas no exact formula translates the degree of suffering into a monetary amount for noneconomic damages. Proof of noneconomic damages depends heavily on the sympathy of the jury or the judge.

The Anatomy of a Lawsuit

The best way to understand the anatomy of a medical malpractice suit is to follow the course of how an actual case would proceed. The case usually begins when a dissatisfied patient walks into an attorney's office with a complaint about a doctor.[8] Occasionally the patient-athlete will complain that a doctor did something wrong or failed to do something she should have done.[8] For whatever reason, the patient is unhappy and feels therefore that someone should take the blame.

Experts

If the attorney feels the case is worth evaluating, he will usually contact a medical malpractice expert to review the case for its merits. The expert may be an attorney who is well versed in medical malpractice actions or, more typically, a physician in the same specialty area as the physician being sued. Often the physicians that review the case to see if it merits filing a lawsuit will be used as the experts to testify if the lawsuit is filed and it reaches court.

Some states have restricted the types of experts that can be witnesses and testify in the courtroom.[9] In the past, regulation of experts was primarily left to the discretion of the court; however, many new state statutes may mean more uniform standards.[3] In addition, some states require expert witnesses to be actively practicing in the specialties in which they testify[10] to deter so-called hired guns who make most, if not all, of their living by testifying in court.[11]

The Petition

If the plaintiff's attorney decides to go ahead with the case after the expert has reviewed it, she will draw up a petition. A petition, also known as the complaint, is a legal document that states how and why the physician, hospital, or other health care provider is thought to be liable.[7] The petition is written in technical and legal terms and phrases that often cause the physician being sued to panic. A sample petition is contained at the end of this chapter, page 26.

Keep in mind that the content of the petition is primarily legal terms that have no actual bearing on what was done or on the outcome of the case. Plaintiffs' attorneys typically delineate any possible allegation in the petitions for fear of leaving an allegation out and then being unable to sue on it later. The petition is usually filed with the County Court and then subsequently "served" on the defendant named in the lawsuit (the physician).

Being served the petition or complaint may be the first indication a practicing team physician has that a lawsuit has been filed. However, there may be hints beforehand that a former or current patient is thinking about filing a lawsuit. The patient may leave the physician's practice to be treated by a different physician or request that his records be copied and sent to an attorney or another physician.

Serving a physician with a petition or complaint is called service of process.[7] This is the official method of serving a defendant physician with a copy of the petition and can be accomplished in one of several ways, which are determined by each state.[7] Frequently a sheriff delivers the document to the physician's home address or office to serve process.

Development of the Defense

If a team physician has any inkling that a lawsuit will be filed or is being filed against her, she should notify the medical malpractice insurance carrier immediately. The team physician should expect to feel panic-stricken and angry when notified that a suit has been filed, but she shouldn't let these feelings delay her from contacting her medical malpractice insurance carrier. The carrier will provide a defense attorney, and the defense of the case can then begin.

The first step in defending the case is to review the records completely. The physician should gather and copy all records pertaining to the case. Although the physician can make notations on copies of the records, in no case should the original records be altered, destroyed, or otherwise modified. The team physician should assist the attorney in delineating what the standard of care is or should have been in the case and help the attorney research the law and medical aspects of the case.

Interrogatories

The next step of the case is to use interrogatories, written questions that are sent to the opposing part and returned with written responses. In medical malpractice, the written questions are directed to the defendant physician.[7] Interrogatories are helpful to establish known facts and to obtain fundamental information.[7] They may help to establish where a doctor is employed, who was involved in the care of the patient, where a physician went to medical school, and other basic information. Interrogatories are an inexpensive method of discovery and are binding on the person giving the answers—in other words, interrogatories may be introduced as evidence at trial.[13]

Depositions

Pretrial oral depositions are also used to elicit information prior to the trial. As with interrogatories, the information obtained from a deposition is binding. Deposition questions typically are more involved and more pertinent to the issues surrounding the case than the questions asked in interrogatories. Depositions, unlike interrogatories, are oral questions and answers recorded by a court reporter. Too often physicians do not prepare adequately for a deposition and thus do not present themselves well. Remember that because 19 of every 20 medical malpractice cases are disposed of prior to trial, the deposition is vitally important—indeed, often decisive.[13] Defendants in a medical malpractice case should thoroughly and adequately prepare for the deposition with their attorneys. Defense attorneys usually can determine what type of questions are going to be asked at the deposition and prepare oral answers to use in the deposition testimony.

Depositions do not have to be taken at any specific place; the defendant lawyer's office, the plaintiff lawyer's office, the physician's office, or a neutral location such as a hotel conference room may be used. Usually, however, depositions should not take place at the physician's office because of the potential for distractions.[7]

Present at the deposition will be the plaintiff's attorney, the defense attorney, the individual being deposed, and a court reporter.[7] The court reporter will administer an oath to the person testifying, who is referred to as the person being deposed. Some states now allow video depositions to be taken.[14]

During the deposition the plaintiff's lawyer will ask the defendant questions. Usually the defense lawyer does not ask questions, because there is no reason to let the plaintiff's attorney know what the defense strategy is going to be, which may occur if questions are asked.

Objections can be made at depositions, but there is no judge there to rule on them. If a statement from a deposition is later brought up in the courtroom, then either attorney can raise an objection and the judge can rule on the issue involved.[15]

The important of depositions cannot be overemphasized. Physicians should prepare for depositions as well as they prepare for an actual court trial. Remember, depositions are taken to discover facts about the case— facts upon which experts will base the case, facts that box in individuals when they testify, and, finally, facts that determine if a case should be settled.[16]

The Trial

The trial is different from a deposition. Observers, the judge, a jury, and many attorneys may be present. In addition, a court reporter takes down virtually every word uttered during the trial. Going to trial is a scary proposition for anyone. It helps to remember that the chance of actually going to trial for medical malpractice is minimal: 90% to 99% of such cases are disposed of before the trial stage.[12]

The trial of a medical malpractice case opens with the impaneling of the jury, if a jury is to decide the case. In many states either side may elect whether a judge or a jury will rule on the issues of the case. After the jury is chosen, the plaintiff's attorney makes an opening statement, identifying for the jury what evidence the plaintiff expects to prove. Following the plaintiff's opening statement, the defense counsel makes an opening statement on behalf of the defendant. Typically this statement explains how the evidence will show that the jury should not render any verdict against the defendant physician.[13]

During the trial the plaintiff has the burden of proving that the defendant is negligent under the law. Thus, the plaintiff presents her case first. The plaintiff's attorney will call witnesses to the stand for questioning, known as direct examination. After the direct examination, the defense attorney cross-examines each witness. Redirect and recross-examinations and further exploration of matters that emerge from testimony can follow. Opposing attorneys can challenge objectionable questions and answers for ruling by the trial justice. A court reporter transcribes all testimony word for word so an official transcript can be made later if needed.[13] Nontestimonial evidence such as medical records, X rays, and reports may be offered by either the defense counsel or the plaintiff's counsel; if accepted by the court, it is entered as evidence and marked so the jury can study it further.

Settlement Before or During the Trial

Most medical malpractice cases are resolved before reaching the trial stage. Claims may be dropped because they were frivolous in the first place. Claims may also be settled with no money changing hands, or claims may be settled when the plaintiff agrees to a settlement offer by the physician's attorney. (It is important to remember that if a settlement offer is accepted and money exchanges hands, the physician's name will be reported to the National Practitioner Data Bank.[3]) In addition, a claim may be settled even after the trial starts. Many considerations influence the decision to settle— even if the defendant has clearly acted in a nonnegligent manner. One is the cost of mounting a defense; others include potential embarrassment, emotional trauma, and lost time due to a lawsuit going to trial.

Practical Considerations

The central issue of all medical malpractice cases is this: "Did the physician act the way a reasonably prudent physician would have acted in the same or similar circumstances?" In other words, what would a physician who is competent in the field of sports medicine have done in the same or similar circumstances? If what the team physician did was what a reasonably competent team physician would have done, then the team physician will not be found to be negligent. Whether there are different methods of treating, evaluating, or rehabilitating the injury that is at the basis of the lawsuit doesn't matter. As long as a certain number of physicians, known as a school of thought, would have acted in the same or similar manner in the same or similar circumstances, the team physician will not be found to be liable.

Practically speaking, most physicians will be sued at some time or other in their professional lives. However, it is uncommon for physicians to have to go to trial. Less than 10% of all medical malpractice lawsuits filed against physicians ever make it to trial. Of these, physicians are found to be liable in only 2% of them. It is even a greater rarity for team physicians to be sued for negligence. This does not excuse the team physicians from practicing competently, however; like all other physicians practicing medicine, team physicians should attempt to be competent in their delivery of care.

All physicians who face a lawsuit go through periods of emotional trauma, which have been compared to the trauma experienced by someone who is facing death. Anger, denial, fear, and depression are common and should be expected.

Physicians who have been notified that they are being sued should contact their medical malpractice insurance carriers immediately. Defense attorneys are experienced with people who are being sued and can help physicians face the emotional trauma of a suit. It's better for physicians to communicate with their attorneys than with other physicians about the issues of a suit—such communication sometimes is admissible in court and can be used against the defendant physician. Team physicians should work closely with their defense attorneys; together they can prepare an adequate and complete defense to a medical malpractice action.

IN THE CIRCUIT COURT OF ANY COUNTY, U.S.A.
at Anywhere

Jane S
100 Anywhere St.
Anywhere, USA 00000,
                              Plaintiff,

v.

Manny M. Moe, M.D.
Anywhere Medical Center South
200 Anywhere Road
Anywhere, USA 00000,

JOHN DOES and JANE DOES
Representing those unknown
parties as described in
Paragraph 3 of this Petition,
                              Defendants.

Case No. _____

PETITION FOR MEDICAL MALPRACTICE

COME NOW Plaintiff, Jane S, by and through her attorneys, I. Jones and O. Smith, and for her claims and causes of action against Defendant Manny M. Moe, M.D., and JOHN DOES and JANE DOES, and each of them, allege and state as follows:

ALLEGATIONS COMMON TO ALL COUNTS

Plaintiff

1. That Plaintiff Jane S is an individual citizen and resident of Any County, U.S.A.

DEFENDANTS

2. That Defendant Manny M. Moe, M.D. (hereinafter referred to as "Defendant Moe"), is and was at all relevant times hereinafter mentioned a Health Care Provider, a licensed physician engaging in the practice of medicine, representing and holding himself out to the public as a specialist in the field of general surgery at Anywhere Medical Center North, 200 Anywhere Road, Any County, U.S.A.

3. That Defendants JOHN DOES and JANE DOES (hereinafter referred to as "Defendants DOES") are named to represent those individuals, agents,

servants, and/or employees of Defendant Moe, named herein above, who were acting within the course and scope of their agency/employment with said Defendant at all pertinent times hereto and whose names are not known to Plaintiff at the present time.

JURISDICTION AND VENUE

4. That the acts hereinafter mentioned giving rise to this cause of action all took place in Any County, U.S.A., and that the causes of action alleged are torts; that the amount claimed by Plaintiff is in excess of $15,000.00; and that pursuant to Section 506.500 R.S.Mo. and Section 508.010(6) R.S.Mo., this Court has jurisdiction and venue, respectively, in this cause.

5. That the relationship of Health Care Provider and patient existed between Plaintiff Jane S and the Defendants, and each of them, commencing on or about January 25, 1991.

FACTS OF THE OCCURRENCE

6. That on or about January 25, 1991, Defendant Moe examined Plaintiff Jane S, with a resulting assessment of fractured right humerus.

7. That on or about February 1, 1991, Plaintiff Jane S was admitted to Anywhere Medical Center North with a diagnosis of fractured right humerus.

8 That on or about February 1, 1991, Defendant Moe performed a left open reduction and internal fixation of the left humerus on Plaintiff Jane S.

9. That Plaintiff Jane S' postoperative course included, but was not limited to, right arm pain, left arm pain, loss of right arm strength and loss of function of the right arm, and problems with a fever of unknown origin.

10. That on or about February 6, 1991, Plaintiff Jane S was discharged from Anywhere Medical Center North.

11. That Plaintiff Jane S continued to have postdischarge problems that included, but were not limited to, right arm pain, left arm pain, loss of right arm strength, and loss of function of the right arm.

12. That on or about February 10, 1991, Plaintiff Jane S was readmitted to Anywhere Medical Center North, where she was diagnosed with the surgical fixation of the wrong arm.

13. That on or about February 11, 1991, Plaintiff Jane S was transferred to Anywhere Medical Center South.

14. That Plaintiff Jane S had a right open reduction and internal fixation of the right humerus on February 12, 1991.

15. That Plaintiff Jane S had to undergo additional medical treatment and follow-up.

COUNT ONE
NEGLIGENCE AGAINST DEFENDANT M. MOE, M.D.

COMES NOW Plaintiff and for her claims and cause of action on Count One of this Petition for Damages against Defendant Moe and Defendants DOES, alleges and states as follows:

16. Plaintiff hereby incorporates by reference Paragraphs 1 through 15 of this Petition for Damages, as though fully set forth herein.

17. That the various and sundry treatment, advice, and counsel rendered by Defendant Moe and Defendants DOES to Plaintiff Jane S, as aforementioned, was careless and negligent in any of the following respects, or all of the following respects, to-wit:

a. In not properly performing the right open reduction and internal fixation of the right humerus;

b. In not obtaining adequate visual field during the open reduction and internal fixation of the left humerus;

c. In not identifying structures properly during the open reduction and internal fixation of the left humerous, including, but not limited to, the side of the body being operated on;

d. In operating on the wrong arm;

e. In failing to diagnose the fixation of the wrong arm;

f. In inadequate follow-up of Plaintiff Jane S after surgery;

g. In failing to timely diagnose and/or properly treat the fixation of the wrong arm;

h. In discharging Plaintiff Jane S without properly diagnosing her illnesses;

i. In failing to order appropriate tests designed to determine whether Plaintiff Jane S had been properly treated;

j. In failing to clinically monitor Plaintiff Jane S;

k. In failing to immediately institute appropriate care and treatment to Plaintiff Jane S for the fixation of the wrong arm;

l. In failing to recognize that the improper surgery had been performed;

m. In ordering the left side of the patient to be draped;

n. In various and sundry other respects that are presently unknown to Plaintiff, but that Plaintiff verily believes will be revealed during the discovery process;

o. In failing to exercise that degree of skill and learning normally exercised by members of the profession of Defendant Moe and Defendants DOES in the treatment of Plaintiff Jane S' condition.

PLAINTIFF JANE S' INJURIES AND DAMAGES

18.   That as a direct and proximate result of the carelessness and negligence of Defendant Moe and Defendants DOES, as aforementioned, Plaintiff Jane S received the following severe, permanent, and progressive injuries, to-wit:

a. That Plaintiff Jane S has in the past and will in the future continue to suffer great physical pain and mental anguish;

b. That Plaintiff Jane S has experienced tremendous psychological consequences as a result of her physical injuries;

c. That Plaintiff Jane S has in the past and will in the future experience loss of sleep and loss of life's enjoyments;

d. That Plaintiff Jane S has in the past and will in the future continue to incur substantial medical, hospital, and prescriptive expenses as a result of her injuries, the exact amount of which is not known to Plaintiff at the present time;

e. That, further, Plaintiff Jane S' ability to work and enjoy life has in the past and will in the future be greatly impaired and diminished;

f. That Plaintiff Jane S has been subjected to unnecessary surgeries as a result of the negligence and trauma inflicted on her by Defendant Moe and Defendants DOES, causing her to incur additional medical and hospital bills;

g. That Plaintiff Jane S may, in the future, be subjected to more surgery as a result of the negligence and trauma inflicted on her by Defendant Moe and Defendants DOES;

h. As a result of the foregoing injuries, all of which were a direct and proximate result of the negligence of Defendants Moe and Defendants DOES, as aforementioned, Plaintiff has been damaged in a sum which exceeds $15,000.00.

WHEREFORE, Plaintiff prays for judgment against Defendant Moe and Defendants DOES, on Count One of this Petition for Damages in an amount that is fair and reasonable as determined by either the Court and/or a jury and those damages permitted by law; for Plaintiff's costs herein expended and incurred, and for such further and other relief as the Court deems just and proper under the premises.

> Jones & Smith, P.C.
> Suite 000, 9999 Anywhere
> Anywhere, U.S.A. 00000
> (000) 555-5000; FAX 555-5001
>
> By: ————————————————
>   I. Jones #00001
>   A. Smith #00002
>   ATTORNEYS for Plaintiff

JURY DEMAND

Plaintiff HEREBY REQUESTS A JURY TRIAL IN THE ABOVE-CAP-
TIONED CAUSE IN ACCORDANCE WITH THE LAW OF THE STATE
OF ANYWHERE.

I. Smith

References

1. *Risk management and the family physician* (2nd ed.). (Not yet released.)
   American Academy of Family Physicians Monograph.
2. Holoweiko, M. (1992, August). What are your greatest malpractice
   risks? *Medical Economics,* **69**(16), 141-160, 141-146.
3. American Medical Association. (1990). *Grand rounds on medical malpractice* (pp. 50-51, 46-61, 58, 303). Chicago: Author.
4. Lyons v. Grether, 239 S.E. 2d 103.
5. Younger, I. (1988). *The advocates desk book.* (p. 333). Clifton, NJ: Prentice
   Hall Law & Business.
6. Missouri Supreme Court Committee of Jury Instructions. (1991). *Missouri Approved Jury Instructions (MAI)* (4th ed.). St. Paul: West.
7. Friedenthal, J.H. (1985). *Civil procedure horn book series* (pp. 270-274, 278-
   280, 168-172, 395, 397, 400, 401). St. Paul: West.
8. Williams, L.E. *Medical malpractice* (Vol. 1, 5.05). New York: Mathew
   Bender.
9. Kansas Statute 60-3413. K.S.A. 185 Supp. 60-3401 and amendments
   thereto.
10. Wisker v. Hart, 168 Kan. 198, 174, 766 P.2d.
11. Roddey-Holder, A. (1978). *Medical malpractice law* (2nd ed.) (p. 405).
    New York: Wylie Medical Publishers.
12. Rumsey, D.L. (Ed.) (1986). *Master advocates handbook* (pp. 51-52). South
    Bend, IN: National Institute for Trial Advocacy.
13. Danner, D. (1986). *Medical malpractice: A primer for physicians.* Roches-
    ter, NY: The Lawyers Cooperative Publishing Company.
14. Missouri rules for civil procedure 57.0376 [videotape].
15. Federal rules for civil procedure, rule 26B1.
16. Danner, D. (1985). *Pattern discovery: Medical malpractice* (2nd ed.) (pp.
    978-980). Rochester, NY: The Lawyers Cooperative.

CHAPTER 3

Are You a Good Samaritan?

A high school has had a contract with a local clinic to provide a team physician at high school football games for years. The team physician is not paid for attending the games, but his expenses are reimbursed. During a Friday-night football game, a safety lowers his head and makes a touchdown-saving tackle on an advancing running back. After the tackle the safety does not get up and complains that he has no feeling in his arms and legs. The team physician runs out on the field and directs the trainers and student trainers in log-rolling the athlete onto a stretcher and into a waiting ambulance. The team physician accompanies the athlete in the ambulance and when the athlete starts to have difficulty breathing, the physician removes his helmet and administers CPR. The athlete is eventually resuscitated in the hospital emergency room, admitted, and diagnosed with a transected spinal cord due to a C-spine fracture.

Questions:

- Is the team physician protected from being sued under a state Good Samaritan statute?
- Does that Good Samaritan protection extend to his treatment of the athlete in the ambulance? At the hospital?
- Does the fact that the team physician receives reimbursement for expenses remove the protection of the Good Samaritan statute?

Many team physicians volunteer their time and effort to local school teams and to other athletic programs. This volunteer participation by team physicians is an extremely valuable service. However, some physicians hesitate to provide care for teams because of their fear of potential liability. In the past 30 years there have been three separate liability crises in which the frequency and severity of lawsuits skyrocketed.[1] Recent surveys show that although claim frequency and damage awards leveled off in the late 1980s, they are now beginning to rise again and it looks as though another liability crisis is looming.[1]

To encourage physicians to continue to volunteer as team physicians, many state legislatures have enacted Good Samaritan statutes that protect physicians who voluntarily provide their services as team physicians from liability.

The History of Good Samaritan Statutes

As defined by a legal dictionary, a Good Samaritan is "someone who unselfishly comes to the assistance of another—a rescuer, humanitarian, helper, aider."[2] Since 1959 all states and the District of Columbia have enacted some type of Good Samaritan statute. These laws vary widely, in both whom they apply to and under what circumstances.[3] The original intent of Good Samaritan statutes was to confer immunity on people who voluntarily acted as "rescuers" to others in distress—it shielded those who altruistically came to the aid of another from subsequently being sued by the individual they rescued. Without such protection the rescuer could be held liable for any negligent act associated with the rescue. This possible liability discouraged people who otherwise would have gone to the aid of someone in peril.[3]

In general, no one has a legal duty to come to the aid of another, unless there is a preexisting relationship that creates a duty. In other words, a woman who happens to be a mother has no duty to rescue a child in danger unless that child is her own. If the child is her own, the preexisting relationship creates a duty in the mother. A physician has no duty to treat anyone except for those with whom she already has a physician-patient relationship. This physician-patient relationship has to be established before the physician has a duty to act.

Only two states, Vermont and Minnesota, impose a duty to rescue persons without a preexisting relationship. However, the absence of a legal obligation to come to the aid of another doesn't preclude a moral obligation. An individual may have no legal duty whatsoever to attempt to save a drowning victim but may feel a profound moral obligation to make an attempt. Physicians have no duty to treat individuals with whom they do not have a doctor-patient relationship, but they may feel a moral or ethical obligation.

Once an individual elects to act as a rescuer to another, then the rescuer has a duty to act as a "reasonable man in the same or similar circumstances."[4] This is the standard in the legal theory of negligence outlined in chapter 2. The possibility of being sued on the basis of not meeting this standard has a "chilling" effect on the actions of rescuers; it causes some individuals who otherwise would have aided another individual to elect to "look the other way."

The classic example of the deterrent effects of the "reasonable man" standard is when an individual comes upon an automobile accident and sees a passenger trapped in the car. The potential rescuer may deliberate whether or not to help the trapped passenger get out of the car. If the person driving by is a physician she may be concerned about the possibility of a cervical fracture in the trapped passenger. Even if there's danger of the car catching on fire, she may worry about potential liability for moving a victim who may be at risk for developing a transected spinal cord. If she moves the passenger, the passenger could later say "but for the physician moving me, I would not be quadriplegic" and sue her. This concern could cause the physician to drive by the accident and not aid the victim at all.

To avoid such a situation, in 1959 California enacted the first Good Samaritan statute, which provided a measure of protection to Good Samaritans, specifically Good Samaritan physicians. Now all states have similar Good Samaritan legislation based on the legislative theory that promoting physician involvement at emergency scenes takes priority over a victim's right to sue. After all, the victim's right to initiate legal action cannot be more important than receiving life-sustaining medical attention, and the former is often dependent upon the latter.[5] Thus, the primary impetus for such legislation is to appease the fears of physicians and to stimulate involvement at emergency scenes.[3]

Current Status of Good Samaritan Legislation

Typically, there are five components of Good Samaritan legislation: the class of persons protected, the requirement of good faith, the standards of conduct, the site of the rescue, and the requirement of gratuitous conduct. Few statutes contain all five components, but all contain at least two.[6]

The Class of Persons Protected

Approximately two thirds of all Good Samaritan statutes grant immunity from civil liability to *anyone* who renders assistance, and thus then protect physicians along with everyone else. Other state statutes specify the classes of individuals who are protected, including physicians, nurses, paramedics, individuals who perform CPR, dentists, and midwives, among others.

Good Faith Requirement

The majority of the statutes require the rescuer to act in "good faith." A California court has defined this nebulous concept as what "in common usage has a well-defined and generally understood meaning, being ordinarily used to describe that state of mind denoting honesty of purpose, freedom from intention to defraud, and, generally speaking, being faithful to one's duty or obligation."[7]

Specific Standards of Conduct

Although most statutes protect rescuers from being sued for negligence, they usually contain some standard of conduct against which the rescuer's conduct will be measured. To avoid liability, a Good Samaritan typically must avoid falling below the standard set by the jurisdiction in which he is acting. Usually, the statutes define the standard of care as the minimum acceptable standard of conduct and use such words as *reckless, wanton, willful, gross,* and *intentional,* to describe conduct that does not meet the standard of care. Rescuers usually will not be liable for any act arising out of the rescue unless their conduct can be characterized as a conscious disregard of the consequences of their actions or a reckless disregard for the rights or safety of others.[8] This is much more difficult to prove in court than ordinary negligence, and, thus, statutes that contain this language confer almost complete immunity for conduct associated with being a Good Samaritan.

However, under statutes in a few states the rescuer's conduct has to conform to the conduct of the "reasonable prudent rescuer in the same or similar circumstances"—the common law reasonable man standard.[9] If a statute contains this language, then Good Samaritans are afforded no more protection than under the laws of negligence discussed in chapter 2.

Site of the Rescue

Most Good Samaritan statutes restrict coverage to the "scene of the emergency."[4] The California statute defines 10 emergency scenes and many other states specifically define emergency scenes instead of using global language such as "scene of the emergency."[10] Such specifically defined emergency scenes are such places as boating accidents, auto accidents, sporting events, outside emergency facilities, coal mines, restaurants, transportation to hospitals, and public gatherings. Some states will even cover a rescuer who acts in an emergency in a hospital.[4]

The Requirement of Gratuitous Assistance

Most states require the Good Samaritan statute to provide assistance gratuitously. To later bill for the care rendered may invalidate Good Samaritan protection.

The Evolution to Sports-Specific Good Samaritan Legislation

Good Samaritan statutes are enacted by the legislatures of various states to encourage physicians to provide emergency assistance. As discussed, physicians, fearing potential liability, may hesitate or refuse to act as a team physician. Recognizing this, some legislators have begun to enact sports-specific Good Samaritan legislation in an effort to allay the fears of team physicians and to promote the voluntary assistance of physicians to sports teams.

Six states have statutes specifying immunity for those who provide their services at an athletic event. These states are Ohio, Kansas, Florida, California, Arkansas, and Maryland. These statutes would protect team physicians.

The absence of a specific statute, however, does not mean that a team physician is unprotected. It is likely that team physicians, acting in an emergency, would still be protected under a general Good Samaritan statute, and, as noted, all 50 states have such statutes.

Team physicians who provide care for athletes in the hospital or in their offices, on the other hand, are usually excluded from the immunity provided by Good Samaritan laws. Sports-specific Good Samaritan statutes usually provide immunity only for care rendered at the sporting event or on the way to the hospital because team physicians who care for athletes in their offices or at the hospital are not subject to the tensions that arise in an emergency situation such as may occur at a sporting event. They have a duty to care for athletes in a competent manner.

What Constitutes Compensation?

In general, compensation is interpreted as the exchange of money from the high school or college to the team physician for provision of care on the sidelines or at practice. Because this exchange of money typically invalidates Good Samaritan protection, team physicians should assure that their contracts specifically state that they don't receive remuneration for providing care.

Many times teams provide team physicians with equipment to be used on the sidelines, transportation to and from games on the team bus or by another mode of transportation, and meals, typically pregame and postgame meals. Usually these extras do not constitute compensation in the legal sense required to invalidate the Good Samaritan statute; more often they are interpreted as expenses that would be incurred by the team physician. Although there is no case law on this point, it is anticipated that courts would find it reasonable for the team to allow the team physician to ride in the team bus or to provide the team physician with equipment for use on the sidelines and not consider this compensation. It is also anticipated that courts would not view the reimbursement of expenses incurred on behalf of the team by the team physician as invalidating Good Samaritan statutes.

The Future of Good Samaritan Laws

Some states, such as Georgia and Maryland, are introducing legislation that also provides immunity for team physicians who provide gratuitous preparticipation physicals.[11] Georgia's legislation, had it been enacted, would have provided that licensed physicians performing physicals for student-athletes or serving as volunteer team doctors would be immune from civil liability.[11] Maryland's recently enacted statute (see page 37) doesn't specifically mention preparticipation sports physical as the Georgia bill did, but the statute appears to cover gratuitous provision of preparticipation examinations.[12]

Physicians have become quite concerned with their potential liability for preparticipation physicals, and some school systems have a difficult time finding physicians to perform them. By enacting such laws, legislators promote the care of teams by physicians by granting them protection from liability for the care that they render.

Practical Considerations

Generally, to be protected under any type of Good Samaritan statute, team physicians must render their services gratuitously. Thus, paid collegiate and professional team physicians are not protected.

The law is unclear whether or not reimbursement for travel costs, free tickets to games for the team physician's family, free meals, and other related monies would be considered compensation and thus invalidate Good Samaritan coverage. What constitutes compensation is usually not clearly defined in the statutes. In general, however, it can be argued that this type of income is reimbursement and not compensation. Team physicians should seek legal counsel about the exact wording of the Good Samaritan statute in the state in which they practice.

Team physicians should execute contracts with the school system or other athletic entity. The contract should clearly specify that the physician is volunteering, for no compensation, her services to the team. More discussion on the clauses that should be included in the team physician's contract can be found in chapter 1.

In general, the uncompensated requirement applies only to care rendered at the site of the emergency—not to care at the hospital or physician's office—and Good Samaritan protection is also limited to any act that occurs at the sporting event. Immunity is usually provided for emergency care of athletes, coaches, referees, and spectators. Some states also grant protection for care rendered to an injured athlete or other individual while on the way to the hospital. In general, though, no statutes protect the physician who continued to treat the athlete in the emergency room of the hospital or at the physician's office. Care rendered in those sites would be measured against the standard of care for negligence. Although preparticipation examinations, treatment of athletes in the physician's office or hospital, and treatment of athletes in the locker room under nonemergency conditions are not covered by the Good Samaritan statutes, the law is evolving toward providing protection for gratuitous preparticipation examinations. Again, physicians should be sure to seek legal counsel about the specific language of the Good Samaritan statute in their states.

Maryland Good Samaritan Statute

The Maryland statute provides:

"s 5-309.4. Liability of volunteer sports program physicians.

- (a) Definitions.
    - (1) In this section the following words have the meaning indicated.
    - (2) "Physician" means any physician, including a doctor of osteopathy, who is licensed to practice medicine in the State.
    - (3) "Sports program" means a program or portion of a program of an institution of higher education or of a public or nonpublic school that is organized for intramural or interschool recreational purposes with activities that include basketball, baseball, football, soccer, track, or any other competitive sports.
    - (4) "Compensation" does not include:
        - (i) Actual and necessary expenses that are incurred by a physician in connection with the services the physician performs for a sports program and are reimbursed; or
        - (ii) The listing without cost to the physician of the physician's name in school or event publication.
- (b) IMMUNITY from liability; exceptions - A PHYSICIAN who voluntarily and without compensation renders services as a PHYSICIAN for a SPORTS program, whether or

not the services are rendered at the request of the school's or institution's administration or a county board of education, is not liable for any damages for any act or omission resulting from the rendering of the services unless the act or omission constitutes:

(1) Willful or wanton misconduct;

(2) Intentionally tortious conduct.

(c) Applicability. - This section shall apply only to:

(1) Treatment at the site of the sports program;

(2) Treatment at any practice or training for the sports program; and

(3) Treatment administered during transportation to or from the sports program, practice, or training.

(d) Scope of section. - This section does not affect, and may not be construed as affecting, any immunities from civil liability or defenses established by any other provision of the Code or by common law to which a volunteer or physician may be entitled."[13]

References

1. Campion, F. (1990). *Grand rounds on medical malpractice* (p. 65). Chicago: American Medical Association.
2. Statsky, W. (1985). *West's legal thesaurus* (p. 352). St. Paul: West.
3. Brandt, E. (1983, Summer). *Akron law review,* **17**(1), 300-392.
4. Mason, R.A. (1987). Good Sam laws—Legal disarray: An update. *Mercer Law Review,* **38**, 1378-1453.
5. Steipel, L. (1981). Good Sams and hospital emergencies, 54 Cal. L. Rev. 417, 434 and n. 107.
6. Mapel, E. (1981). Good Sam laws—Who needs them? 21 S. Texas Law Journal 327, 331.
7. Efron v. Kalmanovits, 249 California App. 2d 187, 57 Cal. Rptr. 248 (1967).
8. Statsky, W. (1985). *West's legal thesaurus* (p. 352). St. Paul: West.
9. Akron. *Good Sam laws: The legal placebo* (p. 320).
10. Cal. Stats. 1976 ch. 824 § 1 currently codified, as amended, at Cal. Bus. and Prof. Code § 2395.
11. Georgia House Bill 1711, introduced 2/17/92.
12. Herbert, D. (1992, October). Reflections on the Gathers case. *Sports Medicine Standards and Malpractice Reporter* 4(4), 58-59.
13. Maryland Statute S 5-309.4.

CHAPTER 4

Athletes and Sport Participation Risks

A star freshman college baseball player is diagnosed with hypertrophic cardiomyopathy and the team physician tells him he must stop playing ball. The athlete, aiming at a professional career in baseball, wants to continue to play. He tells the physician and the college that neither he nor his family will sue if he becomes ill because of participation or if he dies as a result of playing with his condition. The college requires him to sign a release in which the athlete gives up his right to sue the college, team physician, or both if illness or death results from his continued play. During a sprint to first base after a bunt, the athlete collapses and cannot be revived.

Questions:

▌ Are the team physician, the college, or both protected from being sued because the athlete signed the release?

▌ Would the result be the same if the athlete was 17 years old?

▌ Do the answers vary from state to state?

▌ Did the athlete assume the risk of participating after he decided to continue to play baseball even after being told that his participation endangered his life?

▌ Should baseball be considered an inherently dangerous sport?

Team physicians may face lawsuits just as any physician who practices medicine. However, if a team physician is ultimately found liable for negligence, many factors may minimize or abate her liability, including whether she obtained adequate and complete informed consent, whether the athlete assumed the risk of injury that is the basis of the negligence action, whether the athlete executed an exculpatory waiver that takes away the right to sue, whether contributory negligence of the athlete is involved, and whether comparative negligence exists in the state in question.

Informed Consent

Informed consent is a legal doctrine that requires a physician to obtain consent for rendering treatment, performing an operation, or using many diagnostic procedures. Without informed consent, the physician may be held liable for violation of the patient's rights, regardless of whether the treatment was appropriate and rendered with due care.[1]

Development of the Doctrine of Informed Consent

Informed consent has become the touchstone of doctor-patient relations and certainly applies to the team physician. Informed consent arises from the constitutionally derived right of privacy. The landmark *Roe v. Wade*[2] decision deals with the issue of personal autonomy and underlies the doctrine of informed consent.[3] Personal autonomy includes the basic right that individuals may not be "touched" without their permission. An unpermitted touching is a "battery." Thus, if a physician performs a procedure on a patient that was not authorized, that physician could be liable to the patient for a battery.

Most cases regarding consent, however, are based on the question of whether the consent was "informed," that is, whether the provider had given sufficient information about the treatment, including alternatives, to allow the patient to be an informed decision maker.[1] Such cases are usually brought to court on the issue of negligence and not on the issue of battery.[4] A case example appears on page 57.

What Must Be Disclosed

Six items of information must be disclosed to athletes during the informed consent process. These include

- the diagnosis of the patient or athlete,
- the nature and purpose of the proposed treatment,
- the risks and consequences of the proposed treatment,
- possible alternative treatments,
- prognosis if the proposed treatment is not undertaken, and, possibly,
- the cost of the proposed treatment.

Discussing the diagnosis with the athlete is straightforward—the team physician must have some diagnosis in mind or the procedure or treatment in question would not have been mentioned. The athlete must trust the ability of the physician to diagnose correctly to cooperate and undergo the treatment. The working diagnosis is rarely not included in the informed consent process.

The nature and purpose of the proposed treatment also is a straightforward element of the informed consent process. An athlete must understand what he is consenting to have done. Without such information and understanding it can be argued that there is no consent to the treatment, much less informed consent.[3] See page 59 for an early informed consent case.

Disclosing all treatment approaches possible is an additional element of the informed consent process. This area of informed consent is increasingly litigated. In general, the courts have held that all recognized approaches that are reasonably feasible under the circumstances of the particular case should be revealed, if the treatments involve methods the treating physician may be incapable of using or even of evaluating or explaining fully.[5]

The prognosis of the condition and risks of not undergoing the proposed treatment must be fully disclosed to the athlete. This area was highlighted by the infamous *Truman* case in which a patient adamantly and continually refused to undergo a pap smear despite her physician's urging. Ultimately the patient died of cervical carcinoma and her survivors sued the physician based on the physician's failure to inform the patient of the consequences of her refusal. The trial court found the physician liable for the patient's death, but the case was later overturned on appeal.[6] Although Truman was not an athlete, the case law would apply to athletes treated by a team physician.

In these days of heightened interests in cost containment and medical necessity, it is more common for cost—both the physician's fees and the costs of the proposed treatment—to be included in the informed consent process. The informed consent process may also include informing patients of the amount of discomfort they can expect from the proposed procedure. Additionally, some scholars suggest that the informed consent process also include disclosure of financial interests in medical entities to which the patient may be referred.[7]

Standards Measuring Informed Consent

Courts use two standards to determine if adequate informed consent has been afforded the patient-athlete. The most common standard is the physician-based standard: what would a reasonably prudent physician in the same or similar circumstances tell a patient about a procedure or treatment? The key question when using this standard is how to decide how much information is required. Courts have usually held that this is a matter of professional medical judgment.

The second standard, which is somewhat more nebulous, is the "reasonable patient standard." This standard requires that the physician disclose what a reasonable patient in similar circumstances would want to know. This standard was first discussed in the aforementioned case of *Canterbury v. Spence*. In this case the court stated that even if a professional consensus on disclosure did exist, it should not override a patient's right to decide about medical and surgical interventions, a right that could not be exercised effectively unless patients had all the information material to making the decision.[8] The problem with this standard is that what a patient may want to know varies from patient to patient. The area is further confused because courts use two different standards to measure what patients would like to be informed of.

The first of these standards is the *subjective patient standard*, which is based on what the individual patient in question would want to know about a proposed treatment. This standard can be a burden to the physician because it requires knowing the patient in great detail, especially what he would think is important.[3]

An *objective patient standard* relies on what a reasonably prudent patient would desire to know under the same or similar circumstances. Under that standard, physicians trying to determine the scope of informed consent would not necessarily have to take into account individual patient variations. However, some courts have held that even under the objective standard physicians have a duty to inquire about any special fears, values, and sensitivities the patient may have.

State Law Variations

Different states have different laws governing informed consent. A small majority of states have adopted the patient-based approach, with more states adopting the objective patient approach than the subjective one. Other states have adopted the physician-based standard. Some states specify different treatment methods that must be included in any informed consent discussion with patients. As with any other legal doctrine, team physicians should be sure to check with an attorney familiar with the health care laws of their states about the statutory requirements of informed consent. Unfortunately states do not publish books or other material that makes laws on informed consent easily retrievable.

Informed Consent and the Minor

The majority of the athletes team physicians for high school, middle school, and grade school teams will deal with are minors. In general, to adequately make an informed consent, an individual has to have the capacity to consent. Except in limited circumstances, minors do not have this capacity. Hence, team physicians should delay treating minors until parental consent is obtained except in an emergency, when any child of any age can be treated without parental consent.[9] Virtually no lawsuits have been successfully tried solely on the basis of lack of parental consent where the treatment of the minor was nonnegligent.[10]

Many states have enacted legislation known as *minor treatment statutes.* Often these statutes specify an age, usually 16 years but some as young as 14 years, at which a minor is considered completely independent of his parents and able to consent for the purposes of medical treatment. Once again, team physicians should consult with an attorney regarding the specifics of state law.

Emancipated minors are minors who, in the eyes of the law, are completely free from parental control and are self-supporting. These minors usually include married minors and those in the service. Certainly, if faced with an emancipated minor, the physician does not have to delay treatment until parental consent is obtained.

Even in the absence of a statute, many courts are beginning to follow the mature minor rule,[11] which states that if a young person understands the nature of proposed treatment and its risks, if the physician believes that the patient can give the same degree of informed consent as an adult patient, and if the treatment does not involve very serious risks, the young person may validly consent to receiving it.[11]

In addition, the costs of the proposed treatment may be a factor in determining whether the patient is competent to provide effective informed consent. A 15-year-old may be perfectly competent to consent to treatment of acne with a topical antibiotic but may be considered incompetent to consent to treatment with isotretinoin, an expensive antibiotic with potentially serious side effects.

Therefore, to determine if the mature minor rule applies, the physician must consider the treatment contemplated, the age and maturity of the athlete, and the risk of harm. For instance, a 15-year-old may be competent to consent to treatment for a sore throat but may be incompetent to consent for treatment of a metastatic disease.[11]

Fraudulent Concealment

Some cases against team physicians have revolved around intentional fraudulent concealment of information. In *Krueger v. San Francisco 49ers* a professional football player sued the San Francisco 49ers, and one element of the lawsuit was fraud. The Krueger case is discussed in more detail in chapter 6; briefly, however, Krueger was treated for years with steroid and anesthetic injections in his left knee after the San Francisco 49ers and the team physician failed to inform him of the loss of his anterior cruciate ligament. The court in the case held that the 49ers

> consciously failed to make full, meaningful disclosure to Krueger respecting the magnitude of the risk he took in continuing to play . . .

with the profoundly damaged left knee . . . Krueger was in acute pain from 1963 on,. . . he was regularly anesthetized between and during the games, and endured repeated questionable steroid treatments administered by the team physician.[12]

It was clear to the court that Krueger may have made a different decision regarding his ability and desire to continue to play football had he been adequately informed of the risks associated with playing football on a knee that lacked an important ligament and regularly required injections.

Another case involving fraudulent concealment was the case of Michael Robitaille. In this case Robitaille, a hockey player, was hospitalized after suffering an injury to his shoulder and spinal cord. The team physicians concealed the true extent of his injuries, and the team later tried to trade him.[13] The team to which he was traded discovered the extent of his injuries, and Robitaille subsequently sued.

These cases illustrate that team physicians may be liable for fraudulent concealment, the antithesis of informed consent. The legal basis for a suit based on fraudulent concealment is fraud and deceit. The elements of an action for fraud and deceit are

- a misrepresentation or suppression of a material fact,
- knowledge of any falsity,
- intent to induce reliance,
- actual and justifiable reliance, and
- resulting damages.[14]

Team physicians have a duty to fully inform athletes so they or their parents can make informed decisions about the athlete's participation or return to participation following an injury.

Assumption of Risk

An athlete assumes risk when she knows of and appreciates the danger of a given activity and voluntarily chooses to be exposed to the danger.[15] An exculpatory waiver, also known as a prospective release or risk release, is a document executed by the athlete or guardian that releases one party of all or part of its responsibility for another.[16]

Assumption of risk is commonly cited as a defense to a negligence action initiated by an injured athlete. Usually assumption of risk comes into play when the school system or university is named as a plaintiff—it is rarely used when a physician is sued alone. However, it is an important concept for the team physician to understand and will be considered in the context of exculpatory waivers. Team physicians are requiring risk releases or exculpatory waivers more frequently in certain situations.

Express Assumption of Risk and Exculpatory Waivers

Assumption of risk can be express or implied—the former will be discussed here. Express assumption of risk means the athlete or his parents or guardian knew the risk, fully understood it, voluntarily chose to encounter that risk, and agreed in advance not to hold the defendant liable for the consequences of conduct that would ordinarily amount to negligence.[17] Usually this type of case involves a signed document that contains an exculpatory clause, an exculpatory waiver, or a prospective release or risk release. All three terms imply a similar kind of document.

An *exculpatory waiver* or *risk release* is a contract between a participant and an activity instructor or sponsor in which the participant promises not to sue the instructor or sponsor.[18] The purpose of the contract is to relieve the school, university, or team physician from any liability to the individual who executes the contract.[19] Although in the past risk releases usually named only the school or university, they now commonly name team physicians as well. A sample risk release is provided in Figure 4.1. Express assumption of risk can also be effected through an oral agreement.[15]

Abergast v. Board of Education of South New Berlin Central School is an example of express assumption of risk. In that case a student teacher wanted to participate in a donkey basketball game. Prior to participating she was informed of the risk of injury and she expressly agreed to voluntarily participate at her own risk. Subsequently, she was injured in the game and brought a negligence action against the school district. The appeals court held that she was precluded from recovery because she admitted at trial that she had been informed of the risks and voluntarily participated anyway. According to the court, express assumption of risk is a complete defense to a negligence action because when an individual assumes the risk, no duty exists and if no duty exists, no recovery can be made.[20]

Student Information and Parental Approval Form

A. Student Information

1. Student's name _____ Birth date _____ Age ____

2. Name of parent(s) _____

3. Address of parent(s) _____

4. Name of person(s) with whom student resides _____

5. Address of person(s) with whom student resides _____

(continued)

Figure 4.1   A sample risk release form.

6. If this student does not reside with a parent, supply the following information:
   (a) How long has the student resided with this person(s)?_____
   (b) Has a legal guardianship been appointed by the courts?
       Yes ___ No ___
       (If the answer is "yes," submit a certified copy of the court order or letter of guardianship.)

7. School attended last year _____ City _____

8. Grade level completed last June _____

9. Did student pass in at least four (4) full-time subjects in the immediately preceding semester/trimester and receive the maximum credit given? Yes ___ No ___

10. Describe any physical limitations or problems that should be known by the coach:
    _____
    _____

B. Student Rights

Students participating in the Interscholastic Athletic program are governed by the rights, protections, and responsibilities as prescribed by the Interscholastic Activities Association Handbook and their respective schools.

Students and/or their parent(s)/guardian(s) may make application for exceptions to eligibility regulations and may appeal any decisions relative to such requests through their school principal.

C. Student Responsibilities

Participants are required to conform to the rules and regulations of their school and to conduct themselves in a safe and sportsmanlike manner. Violators are subject to probation, suspension, or expulsion.

D. Student Eligibility Requirements

1. Prior to participation in practice of athletic contests a student must:
   (a) have a PHYSICAL EXAMINATION—during the 12-month period prior to first participation in interscholastic athletics in a middle school, a junior high school, and prior to participation in a high school, a student shall undergo a medical examination and be approved for interscholastic athletic competition by a medical authority licensed to perform a physical examination. Prior to each subsequent year of participation a student shall furnish a statement, signed by a medical authority licensed to perform a physical examination, which provides clearance for continued athletic participation.

(continued)

Figure 4.1

The school in which this student is enrolled must have on file a statement (or prepared form) from a medical authority licensed to give a physical examination, certifying that his/her physical condition is adequate for the activity or activities in which he/she participates.

To resume participation following an illness and/or injury serious enough to require medical care, a participating student must present to the school officials a physician's written release.

(b) be covered by the school's athletic injury insurance or have on file in the school office a properly signed League Insurance Waiver form.

(c) have paid for the school's Catastrophic Insurance coverage.

(d) have on file in the school office a signed Student Information and Parental Approval form.

2. To be eligible to participate in an Interscholastic contest a student must:
   (a) be under twenty (20) years of age on September 1 for the Fall sport season; on December 1 for the Winter sport season; and March 1 for the Spring sport season.
   (b) have passed in at least four (4) full-time subjects in the immediately preceding semester/trimester and earned the maximum credit given for each subject.
   (c) be enrolled in and currently passing at least four (4) full credit subjects.
   (d) reside with their parents, the parent with legal custody, or a court-appointed guardian who has acted in such a capacity for a period of 1 year or more.
   (e) not miss practices or games for the purpose of participating in nonschool athletic activities.
   (f) not accept cash awards in any amount or merchandise of more than $100.00 in value, or have ever signed a contract with or played for a professional athletic organization.

3. Students shall be entitled to four (4) consecutive years of participation after entering the ninth (9th) grade.

4. A student completing the highest grade offered in an elementary or middle school is eligible for athletic participation upon entering a public or nonpublic high school. After starting his/her attendance in a high school, a student who transfers voluntarily or involuntarily to another high school shall become ineligible unless he/she obtains a signed Transfer Form from the principal of the high school from which he/she transfers, indicating that the transfer was not for athletic or disciplinary reasons.

5. A student must be in attendance a full day of school on any game date that falls on a school day.

(continued)

Figure 4.1

6. Athletic eligibility can be adversely affected by:
  (a) Providing misleading or false information relative to factors that affect eligibility (loss of minimum of 1 year of eligibility).
  (b) Missing a game or practice to participate in an out-of-school athletic activity.
  (c) Participating in an athletic activity under a false name.
  (d) Engaging in disruptive behavior during practice and/or contests.
  (e) Attending school or practice irregularly.
  (f) Committing and/or aiding or abetting in the commission of any physical abuse or attack upon any person associated with athletic practices or contests.
  (g) Using a school uniform in a nonschool athletic event, failure to properly care for athletic equipment, or failure to return equipment.

We have read, understand, and agree to abide by the Student Rights and Responsibilities and Student Eligibility Requirements listed in this form.

WARNING, AGREEMENT TO OBEY INSTRUCTIONS, RELEASE, ASSUMPTION OF RISK, AND AGREEMENT TO HOLD HARMLESS

(Both the applicant student and a parent or guardian must read carefully and sign.)

SPORT (check applicable box):

☐ Football   ☐ Basketball   ☐ Track
☐ Volleyball   ☐ Wrestling   ☐ Baseball
☐ Cross-Country   ☐ Gymnastics   ☐ Softball
☐ Soccer   ☐ Swimming   ☐ Tennis
☐ Golf

STUDENT

I am aware playing or practicing to play/participate in any sport can be a dangerous activity involving MANY RISKS OF INJURY. I understand that the dangers and risks of playing or practicing to play/participate in the above sport include, but are not limited to, death; serious neck and spinal injuries that may result in complete or partial paralysis; brain damage; serious injury to virtually all internal organs; serious injury to virtually all bones, joints, ligaments, muscles, tendons, and other aspects of the musculoskeletal system; and serious injury or impairment to other aspects of my body, general health, and well-being. I understand that the dangers and risks of playing or practicing to play/participate in the above sport may

Figure 4.1   *(continued)*

result not only in serious injury, but in a serious impairment of my future abilities to earn a living; to engage in other business, social, and recreational activities; and generally to enjoy life.

Because of the dangers of participating in the above sport, I recognize the importance of following coaches' instructions regarding playing techniques, training, and other team rules, etc., and to agree to obey such instructions.

In consideration of the _____ School District permitting me to try out for the _____ High School _____ (sport) team and to engage in all activities related to the team, including, but not limited to, trying out, practicing or playing/participating in that sport, I hereby assume all the risks associated with participation and agree to hold the _____ School District, its employees, agents, representatives, coaches, and volunteers harmless from any and all liability, actions, causes of action, debts, claims, or demands of any kind and nature whatsoever that may arise by or in connection with my participation in any activities related to the _____ High School _____ (sport) team. The terms hereof shall serve as a release and assumption of risk for my heirs, estate, executor, administrator, assignees, and for all members of my family.

PARENT/GUARDIAN

I, _____, am the parent/legal guardian of _____ (student). I have read the above warning and release and understand its terms. I understand that all sports can involve many RISKS OF INJURY, including, but not limited to, those risks outlined above.

In consideration of the _____ School District permitting my child/ward to try out for the _____ High School _____ (sport) team and to engage in all activities related to the team, including, but not limited to, trying out, practicing, or playing/participating in _____ (sport), I hereby agree to hold the _____ School District, its employees, agents, representatives, coaches, and volunteers harmless from any and all liability, actions, causes of action, debts, claims, or demands of every kind and nature whatsoever that may arise by or in connection with participation of my child/ward in any activities related to the _____ High School _____

Figure 4.1

(continued)

(sport) team. The terms hereof shall serve as a release for my heirs, estate, executor, administrator, assignees, and for all members of my family.

The following to be completed only if sport is **football, wrestling, gymnastics,** or **baseball:**

I specifically acknowledge that _____ (sport) is a VIOLENT CONTACT SPORT involving even greater risk of injury than other sports. _____
(initial)

Date: _____ 19 ____ Signed _____
Signature of student

Date: _____ 19 ____ Signed _____
Signature of parent or legal guardian
(if student's age is under 18)

Figure 4.1

Exculpatory Waivers and Risk Releases

Generally, when courts evaluate exculpatory waivers, they weigh the individual's interest in entering into the contract and the interest of protecting the public benefit. In the recent past courts have invalidated exculpatory waivers as a violation of public policy. Public policy violations are based on six different factors:

1. That the agreement concerns an endeavor of a type generally thought suitable for public regulation

2. That the party seeking exculpation is engaged in performing a service of great importance to the public that can be a matter of practical necessity for some members of the public

3. That such party holds itself out as willing to perform this service for any member of the public coming within certain established standards

4. That the party seeking the exculpation possesses a decisive advantage of bargaining strength against any member of the public who seeks the services

5. That in exercising a superior bargaining power, the party confronts the public with a standardized adhesion contract (a take-it-or-leave-it basis) of exculpation and makes no provision whereby those receiving services may pay additional reasonable fees and obtain protection against negligence

6. That the person or members of the public seeking such services must be placed under the control of the furnisher of the services, subject to the risk of carelessness on the part of the furnisher

What the courts are saying by placing exculpatory waivers in the category of public policy violations is that because physicians provide a service to patients and because patients are not usually in a position to refuse that service (they are injured or sick) it would be wrong to let physicians be excused from liability.[21] A case involving waivers appears on page 59.

Many other courts have held that exculpatory waivers are, in general, invalid because they are against public policy.

Although risk releases have been found invalid for many reasons— fraud, public policy considerations, problems with drafting, and even problems with print size[22]—there has been a gradual movement toward upholding risk releases and exculpatory waivers. In these cases the courts have found that the risk release or exculpatory waiver was unambiguous, not against public policy, validly executed, and therefore not unconscionable.[18] To evaluate the validity of the drafting language, the court ascertains whether the language would be "clear to anyone."[18] To evaluate whether the release or waiver is against public policy, the court typically determines if any state law specifically overrides the use of exculpatory and risk releases. Courts my also evaluate whether the right to participate in athletics is in the public policy forum. In other words, should athletes' rights to participate in athletics be protected? Should athletes be allowed the freedom to participate in sports?

What A Risk Release Should Contain

In general, exculpatory waivers and risk releases should be executed in clear, concise, and unambiguous language that any layperson could understand. The release should clearly and explicitly say that it releases the instructor, sponsor, school system, or team physician from liability. It should be printed in a format that is likely to compel any layperson to notice that legal rights are being extinguished. It should be easily readable and should state clearly that it will and can be used in a court of law to demonstrate that the athlete who signs the release understands what it means. The release should note that the person signing it assumes the risk of injuries that may result in death and waives liability for herself or any heirs. It should clearly state what activities are covered under the release and enumerate the risks and hazards to the participant explicitly enough to allow a judge to interpret as a matter of law that the release did contain informed consent.[23] The release should be individualized to the sport in which the athlete wishes to participate, stating clearly any sport-specific risks. And it should be individualized for the athlete—if the athlete has a condition that places him at a higher risk of injury than athletes in general, the condition and the possible consequences of participating should be noted. Finally, the release must be validly signed.

To summarize, exculpatory waivers, also known as risk releases, should inform the athlete of the hazards of participation by specifically enumerating the risks of participation. They should also specifically state that the athlete expressly assumes the risk and waives the right to sue. Waiver forms are contained in Figure 4.2.

WARNING, AGREEMENT TO OBEY INSTRUCTIONS, RELEASE, ASSUMPTION OF RISK, AND AGREEMENT TO HOLD HARMLESS

(Both the applicant student and parent or guardian must read carefully and sign.)

I am aware that tackle football is a violent contact sport and that playing or practicing to play tackle football will be a dangerous activity involving MANY RISKS OF INJURY. I understand that the dangers and risks of playing or practicing to play tackle football include, but are not limited to, death; serious neck and spinal injuries that may result in complete or partial paralysis; brain damage; serious injury to virtually all internal organs; serious injury to virtually all bones, joint, ligaments, muscles, tendons, and other aspects of the musculoskeletal system; and serious injury or impairment to other aspects of my body, general health, and well-being. I understand that the dangers and risks of playing or practicing to play tackle football may result not only in serious injury, but in a serious impairment of my future abilities to earn a living; to engage in other business, social, and recreational activities; and generally to enjoy life.

Because of the dangers of tackle football, I recognize the importance of following coaches' instructions regarding playing techniques, training and other team rules, etc., and agree to obey instructions.

In consideration of the _____ School District permitting me to try out for the _____ High School football team and to engage in all activities related to the team,

Figure 4.2   Sample waiver forms.   *(continued)*

including, but not limited to, trying out, practicing, or playing tackle football, I hereby assume all the risks associated with tackle football and agree to hold the _____ School District, its employees, agents, representatives, coaches, and volunteers harmless from any and all liability, actions, causes of action, debts, claims, or demands of any kind and nature whatsoever which may arise by or in connection with my participation in any activities related to the _____ High School football team. The terms hereof shall serve as a release and assumption of risk for my heirs, estate, executor, administrator, assignees, and for all members of my family.

Date: _____ 19 ____ Signed _____

Signature of student

PARENT/GUARDIAN

I, _____, am the parent/legal guardian of_____(student). I have read the above warning and release and understand its terms. I understand that all sports can involve many RISKS OF INJURY, including, but not limited to, those risks outlined above.

In consideration of the _____ School District permitting my child/ward to try out for the _____ High School _____ tackle football team and to engage in all activities related to the team, including, but not limited to, trying out, practicing, or playing/participating in tackle football, I hereby agree to hold the_____ School District, its employees, agents, representatives, coaches, and volunteers harmless from any and all liability, actions, causes of action, debts, claims, or demands of every kind and nature whatsoever that may arise by or in connection with participation of my child/ward in any activities related to the _____ High School football team. The terms hereof shall serve as a release for my heirs, estate, executor, administrator, assignees, and all members of my family.

Date: _____ 19 ____ Signed _____

Signature of parent or legal guardian

(continued)

Figure 4.2

OFF-SEASON PARTICIPATION CONSENT FORM

The _____ ("Team") hereby grants permission for
          (Team name)

_____ ("Player") to participate in a game or
          (Player)

exhibition of basketball in _____ from (or on)
                                    (Location)

_____ to _____. It is acknowledged that the Player's
   (Date)   (Date)

participation is not part of an NBA or team event. Although the Team's consent for the Player to participate, as required under paragraphs 6 and 17 of the NBA Uniform Player Contract or amendments or modifications thereof, is being given to the Player, such consent is granted solely on the condition that:

> **The player waives any and all liabilities and obligations required of the team under paragraph 6 of the contract or any amendment or modification thereof, and the player further waives any protections or guarantees entitling the player to the payment of salary, bonus and/or deferred compensation under paragraph 2 or 20 of the contract or any amendment or modification thereof, should injuries to the player result from participation in said event.**

The Player understands and acknowledges this waiver. Should any injury occur to keep the Player from playing basketball next season, the Team will not be responsible for paying any medical expenses or for paying the Player's contract that season or any other season for which the Player cannot play basketball.

_____   _____
          Player   Date

_____   _____
      Team Representative   Date

Valid upon Team's receipt of Player's signature.

Figure 4.2

Exculpatory Waivers and Minors

The use of exculpatory waivers and risk releases is becoming more generally acceptable with the adult population. However, with the pediatric population, the population with which most team physicians work, the defenses of assumption of risk and exculpatory waivers have consistently been found in the past to violate public policy.[24]

In addition to violating public policy, assumption of risk and exculpatory waivers are based on contract law, and although minors can legally execute a contract, in most states they are allowed to disavow it any time during their minority or when they reach the age of majority, typically 18 years of age.[25] This means that they may be allowed to act as if the contracts executed on their behalf when they were minors do not apply to them any more.

Courts may not be as ready to allow minors to disavow contracts as they were in the past (as we'll discuss later), but contract law means an added dilemma for team physicians caring for minors. If a minor wants to participate in the sports program despite the team physician's recommendations to the contrary, she cannot execute an exculpatory waiver, and many states do now allow parents to execute this type of contract on behalf of a minor child. Team physicians should ascertain what the law is in their states.

Therefore, even though an exculpatory waiver in general may be allowed, the court may evaluate the validity of a particular exculpatory waiver individually. As discussed elsewhere, if state law precludes the use of exculpatory waivers, team physicians should stand firm and deny the athlete the right to participate in the sport.

Courts May Preclude Athletes From Suing

Even in the face of an invalid exculpatory waiver, courts may consider the subsequent actions of a student and her parents or guardians. The court in *Wagenblast v. Odessa School District*, previously discussed, noted that risks other than the school district's negligence may be present in any athletic activity and if the student knowingly encounters one of these risks and still decides to play, it might be said that the student has voluntarily assumed the risk. The court further elucidated the factors necessary to prove an express assumption of risk. These factors are

1) a full subjective understanding; 2) of the presence and nature of the specific risk; and 3) a voluntary choice to encounter the risk. It is therefore possible that a court would apply the doctrine of assumption of risk, even though the actual waiver form executed may be void as violative of public policy.[26]

Implied Assumption of Risk

More cases have come to court when the assumption of risk was implied than expressed. In implied assumption of risk the consent to assume the risk has not been a matter of express agreement, and a waiver has not been executed. The assumption of risk has been implied from the conduct of the plaintiff under the circumstances.[13] In other words, without an express agreement behavior implies that someone agrees to accept the risk. In implied assumption of risk, three criteria must be met:

1. The injured party had some actual knowledge of the danger.
2. The injured party understood and appreciated the risk.
3. The injured party voluntarily accepted the risk.

The burden of proving that these criteria are met is on the defendant, the school system, or the team physician, and is a matter for the jury to decide.[25]

The team physician encounters the same difficulty with student-athletes with implied assumption of risk as with express assumption of risk. Minors are not held to the same standard of care for their own safety as adults; the standard of care to which they are held may vary with their age and experience.

School districts often use a consent form to prove an implied assumption of risk. In some cases courts have found that consent forms prove the minor and her parents did know of the risks inherent in the sport and agreed to assume them.[27] A consent form will be very useful as evidence that the minor and her parents or guardian were in fact aware of the risks of the sport alluded to on the consent form and elected to participate or allow participation anyway.

However, the consent form, which discusses the risks of the sport, will not eradicate liability that occurs as a result of the school's or team physician's negligence. By signing a consent form, the athlete or his parents only assume the risks inherent in the activity.[28] Thus, if the student's injury was caused by the negligence of the team physician or the school, it did not occur as the result of an ordinary and inherent aspect of the activity, and therefore the consent document would not be helpful to the physician or the school in avoiding liability.[25]

Contributory Negligence

An injured athlete may not be successful in suing a team physician for negligence or recklessness if the athlete is found to be contributorily negligent. *Contributory negligence* is defined as conduct that falls below the standard to which the plaintiff should conform for her own protection and that is a legally contributing cause along with the negligence of the defendant in bringing about the plaintiff's harm.[29] Contributory negligence may arise in sports medicine when an athlete voluntarily decides to take part in an activity and this decision was unreasonable. It may also arise when an athlete deliberately disregards the team physician's warning or instructions and participates in an activity that he was warned against. For example, suppose a member of a basketball team injures his ankle, and the team physician benches the athlete until the ankle is rehabilitated. The team physician warns the athlete not to be involved in any sport activities that involve cutting or other activities that place the ankle at risk. Then suppose the athlete plays a pick-up game of basketball over the weekend. If the athlete injures his ankle during that pick-up game and sues the team physician for that injury, the athlete may be found to have been contributorily negligent because he elected to participate even when the participation was unreasonable. Or if an athlete is given specific instructions on how to put on a piece of protective equipment, ignores those instructions, and then injures the body part that the protective equipment was designed to protect, the athlete may be found to be contributorily negligent because she did not appropriately apply the protective equipment even though adequate and proper instructions were given.

Comparative Negligence

In the past if plaintiffs were found to be contributorily negligent they could not recover damages—the system was all or nothing.[30] Because the theory of contributory negligence seemed so burdensome and unforgiving, courts have gradually begun to use comparative negligence in conjunction with the doctrine of assumption of risk and comparative negligence. Malpractice recovery places the economic loss on the parties in proportion to their fault. If, for example, the team physician is found to be 80% at fault and the athlete who sues the team physician to be 20% at fault, then the athlete will recover only 80% of the damages awarded by the court or the judge.

Practical Considerations

It should be a requirement, as a condition of participation, that each athlete or, in the case of a minor athlete, the athlete's parent execute an informed consent document. The best way to adequately insure that parents and athletes understand what it is they are signing, and thereby consenting to, is to require that the athlete and a parent or guardian attend a team meeting. At this meeting the team physician should be introduced and discuss the sport and its inherent risks. For example, a football team physician should discuss both the serious risks of head injury and neck injury and the less serious injuries such as muscle strains and bruises that are possible in playing football. The team physician should explain that although football equipment has evolved to make the sport much safer than in the past, serious injuries and even death still do occur as a result of participation in the sport. A gymnastic team physician would discuss neck, back, and spinal injuries.

The team physician should also discuss the informed consent document. In general, this document should specifically identify the sport, the most common and most serious injuries that can occur in it, and the team physician. The document should specifically allow the team physician to treat the athlete in an emergent situation, in the locker room after the game, or at practices. In addition, the document should state that the parent or guardian attended the team meeting where the risks of the sport were discussed.

The parent or guardian should be required to sign the document at the meeting. The physician should also sign it, and the athletic trainer or a coach should then witness the document.

The informed consent document is not as exhaustive as a document used in a physician's office or in the hospital setting. It would be impractical, indeed impossible, to include all the risks and benefits of participation in a particular sport in a single document. It is also unnecessary, in light of the relative dearth of cases filed because of lack of informed consent.

By including the most common and the most serious risks inherent in the sport, the informed consent document provides evidence that the athlete and parents knew the risks the sport posed and elected to assume them by choosing to participate or by allowing participation.

This document, if specifically worded, also allows the team physician or athletic trainer to treat the athlete without having to worry about ascertaining her consent status. The document in no way should be construed as forcing the parent to use the team physician as the only health care provider for the athlete. For a variety of reasons many parents want to take their children to health care providers other than the team physician. However, this document will effectively grant the team physician permission to evaluate and treat the athlete in an emergency situation, in the locker room after the game, or during a practice.

If an athlete is injured during the game and is transported to the hospital for care, then the informed consent process will have to be renewed at the health care institution. If the athlete is in a hometown hospital, the parents can elect to have the team physician or the family's own primary care physician care for the athlete. Sometimes the choice may depend on the nature and severity of the athlete's injury or condition.

In general, these preseason informed consent documents should not include waivers of liability or risk releases because many courts would not uphold the validity of an exculpatory or risk release. If an exculpatory waiver or risk release is attached to the informed consent document, it may completely invalidate the informed consent and the team physician who is sued will have lost valuable evidence demonstrating that the athlete and parents were informed about the risks inherent in the sport. However, if the team physician practices in a state where exculpatory waivers have routinely been upheld, he should use them. An example of an exculpatory waiver appears in Figure 4.3.

NOTICE: TO ALL ATHLETES PARTICIPATING IN THE
           INTERCOLLEGIATE ATHLETIC PROGRAM FOR THE
           STATE UNIVERSITY, ATHLETIC DEPARTMENT
FROM: Mr. Friendly, Director of Athletics

_____ is a sport that could cause you serious injury. Participation in the sport is an acceptance of some risk of injury. In order to minimize this risk, it is necessary that you as a participant be aware of and abide by certain safety rules and guidelines.

Any abuse of your equipment or any equipment relating to your sport could cause serious injury to you, your teammates, or your opponents if used improperly.

For example, the football helmet is not be used to butt, ram, or spear an opposing player. This is in violation of NCAA football rules and such use can result in severe head or neck injuries, paralysis, or death to you and possible serious injury to your opponent. No football helmet can prevent all head or neck injuries that a player might receive while participating in football.

Used in a proper manner, all your equipment can be valuable.

You must also report all injuries and any illness to the athletic trainers or team physicians as soon as they become evident to you.

_____

In consideration of the opportunity to participate in the intercollegiate athletic program at the State University during my entire period of eligibility for the program, I hereby certify that I have read and understand the above statement, that I have had an opportunity to ask for explanation or clarification of any portion I did not understand, and that I agree to observe these and other rules and practices that may be employed to minimize my risk of serious injury while pursuing the benefits of this sport.

Signed _____

Date _____

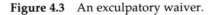

Figure 4.3   An exculpatory waiver.

Most commonly, exculpatory waivers and risk releases are used when an athlete wants to return to participation sooner than the team physician recommends or when an athlete wants to participate in a sports activity against the team physician's recommendation. Both of these situations are discussed more fully in later chapters.

The Salgo Case

The first case specifically citing the doctrine of informed consent occurred in 1957 in *Salgo v. Leland Stanford University Board of Trustees.*[31] The issue in the Salgo case was the nondisclosure to the patient of the risk of paralysis from the performance of a transthoracic aortogram. The Salgo case held that even formal consent documented in writing is legally ineffective if the patient did not understand material information about the procedure being authorized. Material information includes not only the nature of the procedure to be performed but also its broader implications, including any risks connected with it.[32] This case illustrates the point that informed consent is not a document but a *process* of communicating information to the patient, ascertaining that the patient understands the information, and documenting the same.

An Early Informed Consent Case

Most cases related to informed consent have to do with the lack of full disclosure of the risks and consequences of the proposed treatment. According to Rosoff, "A risk is something that might occur in the conduct of, or as a result of, the treatment in question. A consequence is something that is expected to happen."[33] One of the earliest cases on this aspect of informed consent is *Canterbury v. Spence,*[34] in which a 19-year-old male underwent a laminectomy for the relief of low back pain. After the surgery, the patient fell and became partially paralyzed. Although the fall could have caused the paralysis, the patient sued the surgeon, alleging negligence and lack of informed consent. The patient challenged the surgeon's failure to inform him of the 1% risk of paralysis from the laminectomy procedure. The surgeon stated that because the risk was so small, he felt it was in his patient's best interest not to inform him of the risk and that he did not routinely do so. At the appeal level, the court found that every adult person has the right to individual self-determination about health care, and the risk of paralysis may have been material to the patient's decision to undergo the procedure.

Because of this case and cases of similar nature, some physicians are concerned that virtually all risks must be disclosed; however, most courts have held that risks too remote need not be disclosed.[35]

The Wagenblast Case

The Washington Supreme Court applied the public policy test in *Wagenblast v. Odessa School District*. The school district had required all students and their parents or guardians to sign standardized waiver forms as a precondition to each student's participation in athletic activities. The court held that these waivers violated public policy in that

1. interscholastic sports in public schools are a subject fit for public regulation;
2. interscholastic sports in public schools are a matter of public importance;
3. interscholastic sports programs are open to all students who meet certain skill and eligibility requirements;
4. school districts possess a clear and disparate bargaining strength when they insist the waiver be signed;
5. any student who refuses to sign the waiver will be barred from participation in interscholastic sports in public schools; and
6. a school district owes a duty to its students to anticipate reasonably foreseeable dangers.

In addition, the court stated that the school district has a duty to take precautions to protect the students from those dangers, and the student, under the control of a coach, is subject to the risk that the school district will breach its duty.[36]

References

1. American College of Obstetricians and Gynecologists, Department of Professional Liability. (1989). Information for improving risk management. *The Assistants Series* (pp. 13, 17-7), Washington, DC: ACOG.
2. Roe v. Wade, 410 U.S. 113 (1973).
3. Rosoff, A.A. (1991). Treatise of health care law section 17.01 (1). In M.G. MacDonald, R.M. Kaufman, & A.M. Capron (Eds.), *Consent to Medical Treatment*. New York: Mathew Bender.
4. Cobbs v. Grant, 8 Cal. 3d 229, 240, 104 Cal. Rptr. 505, 512, 502 P. 2d 1, 8 (1972).
5. Holt v. Nelson, 11 Wash. App. 230, 523 P.2d 211 (1974).

6. Truman v. Thomas, 27 Cal. 3d 285, 165 Cal. Rptr. 308, 611 P.2d 902 (1980).
7. Informed consent and self referrals. (1989, January). *Family Practice News*, **19**(2), 15-31.
8. Canterbury v. Spence, 464 F.2d 772 (D.C. Cir. 1972).
9. Sullivan v. Montgomery, 279 N.Y.S. 575 (NY 1935).
10. Lacey v. Laird, 139 N.E.2d 25 (Ohio 1956).
11. Holder, A.R. (1978). Minors' rights to consent to medical care. *JAMA*, **257**(24), 3402.
12. Krueger v. San Francisco 49ers et al., 234 Cal. Rptr. at 584.
13. Robitaille v. Vancouver Hockey Club Ltd., 124 D.L.R. 3d 228 (B.C. C.p. App. 1981).
14. Muraoka v. Budget Rent-A-Car, Inc., 160 Cal. App. 3d 374, 414-415 (1983), 196 Cal. Rptr. 117.
15. Statsky, W. (1985). *West's legal thesaurus* (p. 69). St. Paul: West.
16. Appezeller, H. (1985). *Sports and law* (p. 64). Charlottesville, VA: Michie.
17. Keeton, W., Dobbs, D., Keeton, R., & Owen, D. (1987). *Prosser and Keeton on the law of torts* (5th ed.) (p. 482). St. Paul: West.
18. Hulsey v. Elsinore Parachute Center, 168 Cal. App. 3d 333, 214 Cal. Rptr. 194 (1985).
19. Hastings, L. (1988). Playing with liability: The risk release in high risk sports. *California Western Law Review*, **24**, 127-159.
20. Abergast v. Board of Education of South New Berlin Central School, 65 N.Y.S. 2d 161, 490 N.Y.S. 2d 751, 480 N.E. 2d 363 (1985).
21. Tunkl v. Regents of University of Calif., 32 Cal. Rptr. 33, 37-38, 383 P.2d 441, 445-446.
22. Conservatorship of Link v. National Association for Stock Car Auto Racing, 158 Cal. App. 3d 138, 205 Cal. Rptr. 513 (1984).
23. Hastings, L. (1988). Playing with liability: The risk release in high risk sports. *California Western Law Review*, **24**, 153.
24. Henderson, D., Golanda, E.L., & Lee, R. (1991). The use of exculpatory clauses and consent forms by educational institutions. *67 W. Educ. L. Reporter 13* (pp. 14). St. Paul: West.
25. Bjorklan, E.C. (1989). Assumption of risk and its effect on school liability for athletic injuries. *55 W. Educ. L. Reptr. 349* (pp. 367). St. Paul: West.
26. Manno, A. (1990). A high price to compete: The feasibility and effect of waivers used to protect schools from liability for injuries to athletes with high medical risks. *Kentucky Law Journal*, **79**, 867-881.
27. Vendrell v. School District No. 26c Malheur County, 233 Or. 1, 376 P.2d at 409.
28. Kaiser, R.A. (1986). *Liability and law in recreation, park, and sports* (p. 70). Englewood Cliffs, NJ: Prentice Hall.

29. *Restatement of Torts* 2d. Section 281 (1965).
30. Hoffman v. Jones, 280 So. 2d 431, 437 (Fla. 1973).
31. Salgo v. Leland Stanford University Board of Trustees, 154 Cal. App., 2d 560, 317 P.2d 170 (1957).
32. Rosoff, A.A. (1991). Treatise of health care law section 17.01 (1), 17-10. In M.G. MacDonald, R. M. Kaufman, & A.M. Capron, (Eds.), *Consent to Medical Treatment*. New York: Mathew Bender.
33. Rosoff, A.A. (1991). Treatise of health care law section 17.01 (1), 17-14. In M.G. MacDonald, R.M. Kaufman, & A.M. Capron, (Eds.), *Consent to Medical Treatment*. New York: Mathew Bender.
34. Canterbury v. Spense, 464 F.2d 772 (D.C. Cir. 1972).
35. Henderson v. Milobsky, 595 F.2d 654 (D.C. Cir. 1978).
36. Wagenblast v. Odessa School District, 758 P.2d 968, 971-73 (Wash. 1988).

CHAPTER 5

The Preparticipation Examination

Because so many athletes require a preparticipation examination before they can participate in high school athletics, the team physician elects to perform the examinations en masse in the locker room. The team physician has all athletes at the same time rotate their shoulders, squat fully, and bend over and touch their toes. He perfunctorily listens to each athlete's heart and lung sounds. Later in the year a basketball player collapses on the floor. The team physician, with the help of an ambulance crew, resuscitates the athlete but she has suffered an anoxic event and has permanent brain damage.

Questions:

■ Does the locker room type of preparticipation examination expose the team physician to any more liability than a one-on-one examination?

■ Are preparticipation examinations covered by Good Samaritan laws?

■ Is it necessary to perform an examination on a yearly basis?

■ If the athlete had a heart defect that caused her collapse rather than a condition such as a berry aneurysm, would it make a difference in terms of the potential liability of the team physician?

Many states and almost all school systems require a preparticipation sports physical as a prerequisite to participation in interscholastic sport programs. The requirement of the preparticipation examination is an attempt to protect the athlete from injuries caused by a physical condition or defect that could have been discovered during a preseason examination.

The objectives of the preparticipation examination are

- to determine the general health status of the athlete,
- to assess the cardiovascular fitness of the athlete,
- to evaluate preexisting injuries and conditions,
- to assess the athlete's size and maturation,
- to restrict or disqualify the athlete from a specific activity,
- to recommend appropriate activities when specific participation has been restricted, and
- to establish a data base.[1]

The American Medical Association Committee on Medical Aspects of Sports has stated that every athlete has the right to a thorough preseason history and medical evaluation.[2] This statement has imposed a duty on team physicians to provide their athletes with preparticipation examinations and has raised the key legal question of what standard is used to measure preparticipation examinations. The majority of lawsuits stemming from a preparticipation exam allege that the physician performing it did not discover an abnormality that later contributed to an athletic injury. In addition, the new Americans With Disabilities Act and the 1973 Federal Rehabilitation Act affect the team physician's ability to preclude athletes from participation on the basis of a physical abnormality. This chapter will discuss the preparticipation examination in general and the legal ramifications of the exam.

The Preparticipation History

Regardless of what type of preparticipation examination the team physician performs, one of the most important aspects of the exam is obtaining and evaluating a comprehensive medical history of the athlete. The medical history questionnaire should include questions about the athlete's past medical history and past history of sports-related injury. Many, if not all, potentially disqualifying conditions can be elicited by the proper questions on the medical history.[3] A sample history form is contained in Figure 5.1.

All athletes should be required to fill out the history form before undergoing the actual physical part of the examination. If the athlete is a minor, the form should be filled out with the help of a parent or guardian and should be signed by the parent or guardian to ensure that the history is as complete as possible. Some school systems provide forms, which may or may not be comprehensive. If not, consider supplementing them with a form that will provide more information.

History

Name _____ Sex _____ Age _____ Date of birth _____ Date _____

Grade _____ Sport _____

Personal physician _____ Address _____ Physician's phone _____

Explain "Yes" answers below:

	Yes	No
1. Have you ever been hospitalized?	☐	☐
Have you ever had surgery?	☐	☐
2. Are you presently taking any medications or pills?	☐	☐
3. Do you have any allergies (medicine, bees or other stinging insects)? ...	☐	☐
4. Have you ever passed out during or after exercise?	☐	☐
Have you ever been dizzy during or after exercise?	☐	☐
Have you ever had chest pain during or after exercise?	☐	☐
Do you tire more quickly than your friends during exercise?	☐	☐
Have you ever had high blood pressure?	☐	☐
Have you ever been told that you have a heart murmur?	☐	☐
Have you ever had racing of your heart or skipped heartbeats?	☐	☐
Has anyone in your family died of heart problems or a sudden death before age 50? ...	☐	☐
5. Do you have any skin problems (itching, rashes, acne)?	☐	☐
6. Have you ever had a head injury?	☐	☐
Have you ever been knocked out or unconscious?	☐	☐
Have you ever had a seizure?	☐	☐
Have you ever had a stinger, burner, or pinched nerve?	☐	☐
7. Have you ever had heat or muscle cramps?	☐	☐
Have you ever been dizzy or passed out in the heat?	☐	☐
8. Do you have trouble breathing or do you cough during or after activity? ...	☐	☐

(continued)

Figure 5.1 A preparticipation physical evaluation form.

9. Do you use any special equipment (pads, braces, neck rolls, mouth guard, eye guards, etc.)? .... ☐ ☐

10. Have you had any problems with your eyes or vision? .... ☐ ☐

    Do you wear glasses or contacts or protective eye wear? .... ☐ ☐

11. Have you ever sprained/strained, dislocated, fractured, broken, or had repeated swelling or other injuries of
    any bones or joints? .... ☐ ☐

    ☐ Head   ☐ Shoulder   ☐ Thigh   ☐ Neck   ☐ Elbow   ☐ Knee   ☐ Chest
    ☐ Forearm   ☐ Shin/calf ☐ Back   ☐ Wrist   ☐ Ankle   ☐ Hip   ☐ Hand   ☐ Foot

12. Have you had any other medical problems (infectious mononucleosis, diabetes, etc.)? .... ☐ ☐

13. **Have you had a medical problem or injury since your last evaluation?** .... ☐ ☐

14. When was your last tetanus shot? _____

    When was your last measles immunization? _____

15. When was your first menstrual period? _____

    When was your last menstrual period? _____

    What was the longest time between your periods last year? _____

Explain "Yes" answers:

_____

_____

_____

I hereby state that, to the best of my knowledge, my answers to the above questions are correct.

Date _____

Signature of athlete _____

Signature of parent/guardian _____

(Developed by the American Academy of Family Physicians, American Academy of Pediatrics, American Medical Society for Sports Medicine, American Orthopaedic Society for Sports Medicine, and American Osteopathic Academy of Sports Medicine. Copyright © 1992.)

Figure 5.1

Types of Examinations

There are basically three different types of preparticipation physical examinations:

1. Examinations conducted by a personal physician
2. Station examinations of entire teams or groups of athletes during which several physicians each concentrate on a particular area of the body or body system
3. Locker room examinations in which teams of volunteer physicians examine participants en masse[4]

Of the three, the most often recommended is the multistation examination method. This method has been found to be more thorough, and it may result in better detection of potential muscular, skeletal, and orthopedic problems and limitations. The multistation examination also typically results in more recommendations for referrals and further evaluation.[4] On the other hand, some practitioners feel that the doctor's private office is the best setting for a preparticipation examination. They believe that the athlete's personal physician is in the best position to evaluate the athlete, especially if they have a long-standing relationship and the physician is knowledgeable of the athlete's past medical history.[5] The differing perception of the best format for the preparticipation examination is an example of the different standards or practice parameters that exist in medicine, particularly sports medicine, an issue discussed more fully in chapter 1.

Conducting the Multistation Examination

There are several different methods for conducting the multistation type of physical examination. In general this exam uses both ancillary medical personnel and physicians either on-site at the school or in the team physician's office. It is called *multistation* because the athlete proceeds from station to station for evaluation.

Typically, the athlete signs in at the initial station where the history form is reviewed for completeness. It can be helpful to highlight areas of concern on the history form. Seeing highlighted items, the examining physician is more likely to specifically address them. It is essential that personnel at the initial station have the proper training and background to make such determinations. A nurse, physical therapist, athletic trainer, or physician usually fills this role.

At the second station the athlete is weighed, height and blood pressure are measured, and a visual acuity test is performed. It is also helpful to check the athlete's eyes for anisocoria at this station. All of these evaluations can be performed by a nurse or other properly trained individual.

An athlete's musculoskeletal system can be evaluated at the next station, including a check of flexibility. Typically, either a physician or a physical therapist conducts the evaluation.

Evaluating the cardiovascular and lung systems comprises the next station. This part of the examination is performed by a physician, and the environment should be quiet. The physician also examines the skin in a general way, the abdomen, and the genitalia. The athlete's level of maturation is evaluated here as well.[6]

The final part of the examination, the physician's overall assessment of the athlete, can conclude the physical examination or be a separate station. The physician informs the athlete of her recommendations, which may include training guidance, such as flexibility or strength training, or any recommendations stemming from the findings of the history and physical examination. If a physician is going to recommend against clearance, he can discuss that stance with the athlete here. As an alternative the team physician may wish to schedule an appointment with the athlete for a more thorough discussion.

Examinations by Individual Physicians

Advocates of preparticipation examinations by an individual physician usually suggest scheduling 30 min for the examination.[7] This usually allows time to inquire about the athlete's life and home situation and to discuss issues that might be unrelated to the athletic endeavors, such as pregnancy prevention and adolescent health care issues. Arguably, this type of exam allows the physician to devote more time to anticipatory guidance.

"Locker Room" Preparticipation Examinations

"Locker room" physicals or physicals done en masse have fallen into disrepute and probably justifiably so. The examination is usually cursory. It lacks privacy, which precludes any kind of individual counseling. The environment is usually very noisy, making it difficult, if not impossible, to hear an athlete's heart and lung sounds. A reasonably quiet environment is a necessity to pick up subtle cardiac murmurs or arrhythmias that may indicate the presence of underlying disease. For these reasons locker room physicals are potentially dangerous and should be avoided.[8]

The Preparticipation Examination Form

Team physicians use many preparticipation examination forms. Figure 5.2 is a form recommended by the American Academy of Family Physicians, the American Academy of Pediatrics, the American Orthopedic Society for

Physical Examination   Date _____

Name _____

Age _____ Date of birth _____

			Normal	Abnormal findings					Initials
COMPLETE	LIMITED	**Height _____ Weight _____ BP ___ / ___ Pulse _____**							
		Vision R 20/____ L 20/____ Corrected: Y N Pupils _____							
		Cardiopulmonary							
		Pulses							
		Heart							
		Lungs							
		Tanner stage	1	2	3	4	5		
		Skin							
		Abdominal							
		Genitalia							
		Musculoskeletal							
		Neck							
		Shoulder							
		Elbow							
		Wrist							
		Hand							
		Back							
		Knee							
		Ankle							
		Foot							
		Other							

Clearance:

A. Cleared

B. Cleared after completing evaluation/rehabilitation for: _____

C. Not cleared for:

☐ Collision

☐ Contact

☐ Noncontact ____ Strenuous ____ Moderately strenuous ____ Nonstrenuous

Due to: _____

Recommendation: _____

_____

Name of physician _____ Date _____

Address _____ Phone _____

Signature of physician _____

(Developed by the American Academy of Family Physicians, American Academy of Pediatrics
American Medical Society for Sports Medicine, American Orthopaedic Society for Sports
Medicine, and American Osteopathic Academy of Sports Medicine. Copyright © 1992.)

Figure 5.2   A sample preparticipation physical form.

Sports Medicine, the American Medical Society for Sports Medicine, and the American Osteopathic Academy for Sports Medicine. If a school system provides a standardized form, carefully evaluate its adequacy. Many school systems' standardized forms are too short and not inclusive. The team physician may not have the option of whether or not to use the school system's form, but if it is inadequate, use a supplement to keep a thorough preparticipation examination history and physical record.

Recommendations

Regardless of the type of examination performed, certain types of recommendations should result. From the preparticipation examination, a physician can make recommendations regarding conditioning, rehabilitation, and balanced competition.

Proper Conditioning Recommendations

One of the recommendations that should result from the preparticipation exam regards conditioning. This type of anticipatory counseling is especially helpful if the examination is performed some months before the athlete will actually participate in the sport. If the physician identifies a prior injury, he can instruct the athlete in conditioning and rehabilitative exercises specific to the injury. Many athletes, especially male athletes, are relatively inflexible. The physician should provide flexibility exercises for these athletes. Often if they increase flexibility, they decrease the chance of injury.

Proper Rehabilitation Recommendations

Perhaps one of the most important aspects of the preparticipation examination is the opportunity to evaluate past injuries to ascertain if the athlete has been properly and completely rehabilitated before she returns to competition. The carefully designed health history questionnaire will identify special problems such as an unrehabilitated injury, serial concussions, and other injuries or conditions that have a direct impact on participation in certain sports.[9] Performing the physical a few months prior to participation allows the athlete to carry out the proper conditioning and rehabilitative exercises before engaging in competition.

Balanced Competition Recommendations

Another objective of the preparticipation examination is to assess the physical maturity of the athletes. Despite controversy over the usefulness of physical maturity assessment by Tanner staging, such assessment can help assure that participants compete against other athletes who are at a similar maturity level.[10] Age is not a completely satisfactory index of young athletes' physical capabilities. Although no definitive data support the theory, many team physicians feel that immature athletes, those in lower Tanner stages, are at a greater risk for both physical and psychological damage if they compete in collision and contact sports with more mature athletes.[11] Evidence suggests that young athletes are at greatest risk for injury to the musculoskeletal system during their prepubescent growth spurt. Keep this in mind when recommending matching participants, and consider separating pre- and postpubescent athletes to try to reduce injury in contact sports. Make these recommendations not only to the athlete and parents, but also to the school system.

Athletes have sued on the issue of balanced competition. One case involved an inexperienced 130-lb lacrosse player matched against a 260-lb senior with 3 years of experience. During a drill, the younger, inexperienced athlete suffered a broken arm. He subsequently brought suit for his injuries, contending that the school district and coach were responsible because of the mismatching of participants.[12]

Another case involved a high school football player who broke his neck playing in a league game. The athlete who sued was a member of a football team that was transferred into a more competitive division of interscholastic football over the objections of the coach and the school. They had requested a transfer back to the less competitive division because of concerns that participating in the more competitive division would be unsafe. Eventually, the school system and the coaches were found to be liable for the athlete's injuries.[13]

Both of these cases were directed at school systems and coaches; however, the literature does suggest that team physicians evaluate the Tanner stages of participating athletes to properly match them for balanced competition. Because appropriate sports medicine literature makes this recommendation, team physicians may be held liable for injuries sustained by mismatched participants.

Timing and Number of Examinations

How often should sports exams be performed? Sometimes state law determines frequency. Many states require an annual preparticipation exam for all athletes in interscholastic sports at the junior high school and high school levels. Some health care professionals, including primary care physicians, feel that a yearly exam is ideal, especially for adolescents. These professionals feel that a yearly exam is the ideal time to offer anticipatory guidance and evaluate and make recommendations regarding old injuries.[14] Other physicians recommend that the exam be performed less often, commonly every 3 years or with each entry to a new level, for example, at the start of junior high school, high school, and college.[15,16] If this approach is followed, however, it should include a mechanism for evaluating athletes who have been injured the preceding year before allowing them to participate the subsequent year. The American Academy of Pediatrics recommends that a full examination be performed at entry level followed by yearly updates with abbreviated histories and physical examinations.

Areas of Potential Liability

Two topics that warrant discussion regarding liability and the preparticipation examination include failure to diagnose and Good Samaritan statutes.

Failure to Diagnose

Failure to diagnose is the most common allegation against primary care physicians.[17] This is an easily identifiable area of potential liability for the team physician who conducts the preparticipation examination. If the team physician faces a lawsuit alleging that he missed a diagnosis in the preparticipation examination, the forms used, the examination format, the environment, and the scope of the exam will be evaluated by the plaintiff's attorney and subsequently by the court.

Cardiac Anomalies, Arrhythmias, and Sudden Cardiac Death

Some of the most important areas of concern are the proper diagnosis and evaluation of cardiac anomalies. Data for males playing in interscholastic and intercollegiate basketball indicated that the risk of exercise-induced sudden cardiac death is approximately 7 per 100,000 participants per year, a rate that is 14 to 35 times higher than the rate observed for young men exercising in other situations.[18] The risk of cardiac arrest among young adults in general during vigorous exercise has been found to be 5.5 cases per 100,000.[19] The sudden death of Loyola Marymount's star basketball player, Hank Gathers, highlights the importance of proper cardiac evaluation. If an athlete dies suddenly, litigation is sure to follow.

The most common causes of sudden death in athletes are cardiac anomaly, and one of the most common anomalies to cause sudden death is hypertrophic obstructive cardiomyopathy.[20] The risk to athletes with hypertrophic cardiomyopathy who participate in aerobic sports is very high, and these athletes usually are precluded from participation.

Mitral valve prolapse is probably the most common cardiac valve disorder, affecting approximately 5% of the population.[21] Mitral valve prolapse usually is not a contraindication to athletic participation unless the athlete has a history of syncope, disabling chest pain, or complex ventricular arrhythmias, particularly if induced or worsened by exercise; significant mitral regurgitation; prolonged QT interval; Marfan's syndrome; or a family history of sudden death. Information about these conditions should be elicited during the preparticipation examination.[21] Athletes with mitral valve prolapse and a history of one of these conditions that constitutes grounds for exclusion might attempt to use exculpatory waivers to enable them to participate.

Cardiac arrhythmias are another potential basis for recommending that an athlete be excluded from play. Perhaps the most famous example is the Hank Gathers case, in which a star college basketball player for Loyola Marymount collapsed on the court and died.

Hank Gathers suffered from a cardiac arrhythmia. Loyola Marymount's team physician was aware that Gathers had an arrhythmia. In fact, in the weeks prior to his death, Gathers collapsed on the floor while playing.[22] The issues in the case were whether Gathers should have been participating at all and, if so, under what circumstances. The episode of witnessed syncope alone could have been the basis for excluding Gathers from any further participation. But Gathers' desire to pursue an NBA career and his personal love for the game complicated the scenario. Another issue complicating the case is whether, as many news reports suggested, Gathers would have reduced his dose of medication if something other than propranolol, with all its known negative side effects, had been prescribed. A $32.5 million lawsuit was filed by Gathers' family alleging, among other things, wrongful death.[23] The lawsuit was later settled for an undisclosed amount, but it highlights the essential nature of adequate screening for cardiac abnormalities and informed consent.

If a lawsuit does arise after a case of sudden death, the court will evaluate whether the physician performed a cardiac exam and under what circumstances. In addition, if the physician knew the athlete had a condition that might place her at a high risk of sudden death, the court will inquire whether the physician made the proper recommendations or took the proper precautions. Thus, the importance of carefully eliciting the athlete's cardiac history, including information about his family, and carefully performing a cardiac examination cannot be overemphasized.

The discussion of cardiac abnormalities is not complete without discussing the issue of whether widespread screening with noninvasive cardiac technologies should be implemented. Studies indicate that the predominant cause of sudden death in boys and men less than 35-45 years old is due to cardiac structural abnormalities that frequently were not previously suggested by symptom, history, or diagnoses.[24] Nevertheless, the occurrence of cardiac abnormalities in this age group is extremely low in relation to the cost of widespread, noninvasive cardiac evaluation such as ECGs, exercise stress tests, and echocardiograms. Therefore, widespread screening is not indicated.[25]

Controversy remains, however, over different published guidelines and professional standards of care for athletes with cardiac anomalies and arrhythmias. In general, if an athlete has a family history of sudden death or a personal history of witnessed syncope, then the prudent team physician should perform a careful medical examination including noninvasive assessments and invasive screening if indicated. Physician judgment will still determine the depth of the evaluation because the final decision about whether the athlete will be safe participating in sports must be a subjective one.[22]

The National Institutes of Health developed clearly defined recommendations for sports participation by athletes with certain cardiac conditions at the 16th Annual Bethesda Conference. Team physicians should be thoroughly familiar with these recommendations and conform to them.[26]

Diagnosing Other Injuries or Conditions

The allegation of failure to diagnose can also occur if the physician fails to diagnose an old injury or condition, the athlete is then further injured by participating in a sport, and that further injury could have been prevented by proper and timely diagnosis and interventional recommendations. For example, if the physician misses an improperly rehabilitated anterior cruciate injury and the athlete sustains a complete tear of the anterior cruciate participating in sports, the physician could be liable for failing to diagnose the improperly rehabilitated knee, failure to recommend appropriate strengthening exercises, and failure to recommend that the athlete wear some type of supportive brace.

This example illustrates the critical nature of a proper musculoskeletal examination and the necessity of proper and appropriate recommendations. It also illustrates that good risk management—making the proper recommendations—is also good sports medicine. Proper evaluation and recommendations to the athlete help insure that the athlete is able to perform at her best.

The athlete also has a responsibility to report previous injuries to the examining physician. If the athlete fails to report a previous injury and the injury was not easily identifiable during a routine preparticipation exam, then the physician has no responsibility to make any recommendations regarding the injury.

The Preparticipation Examination and Good Samaritan Statutes

In most instances Good Samaritan statutes do not provide immunity for physicians who gratuitously render preparticipation examinations. However, legislatures are beginning to recognize that team physicians are quite concerned about their liability for preparticipation examinations. This concern has increased after the Gathers case. Some legislatures have taken positive actions toward including preparticipation examinations in their Good Samaritan statutes. As we discussed earlier, Georgia recently introduced a bill that would have granted immunity to team physicians from civil liability for rendering physicals to student athletes.[27] Although the bill was not passed, the fact that it was introduced indicates that legislators are considering this issue. As Good Samaritan statutes evolve, more and more will be written to specifically cover team physicians and their provision of preparticipation examinations.

Precluding the Athlete From Participation

One of the reasons for a preparticipation examination is to determine whether an athlete has a condition that may preclude her participation in certain sports. Cardiac anomalies, previous head injuries, the absence of an organ, and previous musculoskeletal injuries may cause a team physician to recommend that the athlete be precluded from participation. In 1988 the American Academy of Pediatrics published the recommendations for participation in competitive sports noted in Figure 5.3. These recommendations provide team physicians with guides to clinical decisions clearing athletes to participate. In addition, the National Institutes of Health has issued recommendations regarding participation of athletes with cardiac conditions.[26]

Precluding an athlete from participating in sports used to be fairly simple and straightforward, but limitations by team physicians have recently been challenged in the courtroom. Athletes have no constitutionally protected right to participate in interscholastic sports. However, in the last 20 years, the federal government has created rules and regulations that guide participation by athletes in sports.

The Federal Rehabilitation Act and the Americans With Disabilities Act

The Federal Rehabilitation Act (9/26/73 29 U.S.C. §701-709, 720-724, 730-732, 740, 741, 750, 760-764, 770-776, 780-787, 790-794, P.L. 93-112) was enacted in 1973. Since then challenges to decisions made by team physicians to exclude athletes from participation in interscholastic or intercollegiate athletics have been made based on the act. To assert a right to participate under the Federal Rehabilitation Act (see page 84), an athlete must prove each of the following elements:

1. That the program or activity in question receives federal assistance
2. That the athlete is an intended beneficiary of the federal assistance
3. That the individual is an "otherwise qualified" handicapped person

	Contact		Noncontact		
	Contact/collision	Limited contact/collision	Strenuous	Moderately strenuous	Nonstrenuous
Atlantoaxial instability *Swimming (no butterfly, breaststroke or diving starts)	No	No	Yes*	Yes	Yes
Acute illnesses *Needs individual assessment (e.g., contagiousness to others, risk of worsening illness)	*	*	*	*	*
Cardiovascular					
Carditis	No	No	No	No	No
Hypertension					
Mild	Yes	Yes	Yes	Yes	Yes
Moderate	*	*	*	*	*
Severe	+	+	+	+	+
Congenital heart disease *Needs individual assessment +Patients with mild forms can be allowed a full range of physical activities; patients with mild or severe forms or who are postoperative should be evaluated by a physician					
Eyes					
Absence or loss of function of one eye	*	*	*	*	*
Detached retina	+	+	+	+	+
*Availability of American Society for Testing Materials approved eye guards may allow competitor to participate in most sports, but this must be judged on an individual basis +Consult ophthalmologist					
Inguinal hernia	Yes	Yes	Yes	Yes	Yes
Kidney (absence of one)	Yes	Yes	Yes	Yes	Yes
Liver (enlarged)	No	No	Yes	Yes	Yes

Figure 5.3   Recommendations for participation in competitive sports.

(continued)

	Contact		Noncontact		
	Contact/ collision	Limited contact/ collision	Strenuous	Moderately strenuous	Nonstrenuous
Musculoskeletal disorders *Needs individual assessment	*	*	*	*	*
Neurologic					
History of serious head or spine trauma, repeated concussions or craniotomy	*	*	Yes	Yes	Yes
Convulsive disorder					
Well controlled	Yes	Yes	Yes	Yes	Yes
Poorly controlled	No	No	Yes+	Yes	Yes++
Ovary (absence of one)	Yes	Yes	Yes	Yes	Yes
Respiratory					
Pulmonary insufficiency	*	*	*	*	Yes
Asthma	Yes	Yes	Yes	Yes	Yes
Sickle cell trait	Yes	Yes	Yes	Yes	Yes
Skin (boils, herpes, impetigo, scabies)	*	*	Yes	Yes	Yes
Spleen (enlarged)	No	No	No	Yes	Yes
Testicle (absent or undescended)	Yes*	Yes*	Yes	Yes	Yes

*Needs individual assessment
†No swimming or weight lifting
††No archery or riflery

*May be allowed to complete if oxygenation remains satisfactory during a graded stress test

*No gymnastics with mats, martial arts, wrestling or contact sports until no longer contagious

*Certain sports may require protective cup

Note. Reproduced by permission of *Pediatrics*, Vol. 81, page 737. Copyright 1988.

Figure 5.3

4. That the individual is being excluded from participation in a program or is denied benefits solely by reason of a handicap[28]

Athletes have been allowed to compete with only one kidney, only one eye, and various other handicaps but only upon showing substantial medical evidence that no risk of further injury exists.[29] The court often gives weight to medical recommendations from physicians, ultimately deciding that the school's concern for the safety of the athlete and for avoiding liability is outweighed by the medical testimony that the athlete can participate.[29]

However, the "otherwise qualified language" of Section 504 of the Rehabilitation Act could be interpreted to mean that the athlete has to have been cleared to participate by at least one physician. If the athlete has not been cleared to participate by a medical expert because of a medical condition or the high likelihood of potentially catastrophic injury, the athlete may be determined not "otherwise qualified," and therefore it may be permissible to bar participation.

This occurred in a case involving a high school football player, Steve Larkin, who sued under the Federal Rehabilitation Act when he was not permitted to play football due to the discovery of a heart defect. The court rejected Larkin's challenge because he did not have a signed medical authorization providing him clearance and had failed to provide a favorable medical opinion. Thus Larkin did not meet the "otherwise qualified" element of Section 504 and could not successfully sue for participation under the Federal Rehabilitation Act.[30] Larkin later went on to play baseball with the Texas Longhorns after executing an exculpatory waiver.

The more recent enactment of the Americans With Disabilities Act (ADA) of 1990 (P.L. 101-336 42 U.S.C. §12101 et seq. & 47 U.S.C. §225 & §611) may also provide a method for athletes to challenge a team physician's decision about participation in athletics. One of the ADA's mandates is to provide a clear and comprehensive national mandate for the elimination of discrimination against individuals with disabilities.[31] The ADA grants people who are physically disabled status as a protected class for purposes of employment, transportation, public accommodation, and telecommunications.[31] Individual athletes may be deemed to be "disabled" or differently abled and thus may be entitled to access to public accommodations. Under the ADA, participation in sports activities may be interpreted as a public accommodation.

The ADA specifies three tests to determine if someone is disabled. One test requires showing that an impairment substantially limits a major life activity. Another test requires a record of the impairment in a preparticipation examination form or a physician's notes and charts. Under the third test, if the general public would perceive that the athlete's impairment limits a major life activity, then the athlete would be deemed to be disabled. Thus, to be covered under the ADA an athlete must meet any one of the three tests: He must have an impairment that substantially limits his major life activities, there must be a record of such an impairment, or the general public would regard him as having such an impairment.

For example, in the case of *Grube v. Bethlehem Area School District* the plaintiff, a high school student with one kidney, sought to enjoin school officials from preventing him from playing football.[32] The court did find the athlete handicapped under the Federal Rehabilitation Act but the athlete might not have been found handicapped under the ADA. The lack of one kidney does not severely restrict the athlete's major life activities compared to most other people, and the ADA has been designed to protect *only* individuals who have handicaps that rise to the level of a "substantial limitation."[31] However, the court may have ultimately determined that the athlete was handicapped under the ADA if there was a record showing he lacked one kidney or if the school officials and others regarded him as being handicapped.

It is difficult to foresee the impact of the ADA on team physicians' decisions to recommend against clearance for participation. The ADA has not been tested in the courtroom.

What these federal enactments underscore is the importance of thoroughly explaining the basis for the recommendation of excluding the athlete from participation. Ultimately choice of whether or not to participate is the athlete's or her parents'. The team physician has a duty to properly inform the patient of the basis for his recommendation so the athlete or her parents can make an informed decision.

Participating Despite the Physician's Recommendation

Athletes are increasingly obsessed with participating, and some have attempted to convince physicians and school systems to allow them to participate by waiving their right to sue.[33] The case of the football player, Steve Larkin, is a good example. Larkin suffers from hypertrophic cardiomyopathy and was precluded from sports participation in his final 2 years of high school. However, through an administrative jumble he played in the starting lineup of the University of Texas baseball team until an administrator heard about his condition and school officials forced him off the field. Finally, his parents signed an exculpatory waiver, which they had offered to do at the time of his enrollment, and Larkin was allowed to play.[33]

The question arises of how informed Larkin is about his condition. Larkin has been quoted in the newspaper as saying that "death can happen if I'm sitting at home watching TV or whether I'm playing." Clearly participating in any cardiovascularly demanding sport places an athlete with hypertrophic cardiomyopathy at a much higher risk of dying than does any sedentary activity.[33]

The Hank Gathers case, discussed previously, also illustrates the difficulties encountered when athletes with potentially disqualifying conditions are identified. Gathers had an arrhythmia that, in the past, would have precluded his participation from sports. Yet he was allowed to participate. Although all the facts of the case have not been released to the general public, it appears that Gathers knew he had a problem and chose to play anyway.[34]

Both cases underscore the crucial nature of informed consent. Both of these athletes needed in-depth counseling regarding the nature of their disorders and the consequences, including death, which they faced by participating in aerobic sports.

Some injuries and conditions have traditionally precluded athletes from participation, but the Federal Rehabilitation Act and the ADA have complicated the situation. If the athlete or his family demand that participation be allowed, consider requiring the athlete to execute an exculpatory waiver. The execution of the waiver must be accompanied by in-depth informed consent, as discussed in chapter 4. In those states that do not enforce exculpatory waivers, stand firm and exclude the athlete from participation. Otherwise, the potential for liability if a tragedy related to the disqualifying condition occurs is enormous. If the athlete pursues a court order to participate under the ADA or the Federal Rehabilitation Act and the court orders that participation be allowed after hearing the rationale for the athlete's preclusion, the court order markedly diminishes and may extinguish the team physician's liability.

If the athlete participates because of a court order or an exculpatory waiver, the team physician has a duty to inform the athlete of available methods to reduce the chance of injury.[35] Knowledge of available protective gear and the risks and consequences of injury associated with different sports is essential in decision making.[35] Instruct single-eyed athletes to wear appropriate protective eye gear, athletes with one kidney to wear extra padding, and athletes with one testicle to wear a protective cup. Even if the team physician disagrees with the athlete's decision to participate, she has the duty of working with the athlete to ensure safety to the extent possible. Team physicians on the sidelines during practices or games in which an athlete is participating after executing an exculpatory waiver or by court order must make all attempts to insure that the athlete is participating as safely as possible, perhaps by the addition of extra equipment or the closer proximity of emergency resuscitation devices. For example, at the Loyola Marymount games in which Hank Gathers participated the team physician had a defibrillator within immediate reach. Each clinical situation must be evaluated individually and recommendations for available equipment and personnel must be uniquely identified.

Practical Considerations

The team physician must first decide on the format for the preparticipation examination—at the school or in the office, with many assistants or working individually with the athletes. Regardless of the format, each athlete must be required to complete a medical history form prior to reporting for the physical exam. Giving the athlete the form before the exam and requiring a parental signature helps ensure that the information on the form is accurate and that parents have read it. If an athlete does not report for the physical with a completed history form, she should not be examined.

The history form should indicate the sport in which the athlete will participate. It should include an entire section devoted to previous injuries, especially previous head injuries and injuries related to heat intolerance. The history form should include a family history and specifically ask about sudden death among relatives. Another section should elicit information about any chronic illnesses such as asthma, diabetes, or hypertension. This information will enable the examining physician to tailor the physical examination to specific problems. For example, if an athlete has sustained a previous injury to a knee, a team physician can more thoroughly examine the knee to evaluate whether it has been completely rehabilitated or whether it might require a brace.

The physical examination should be done in a quiet area where the team physician can adequately hear heart and lung sounds. The physical examination should include evaluation of the musculoskeletal and cardiorespiratory system, an in-depth evaluation with the athlete of his medical history, and a more in-depth evaluation of a particular area if the athlete has sustained any previous injury.

After the preparticipation history and physical examination, the team physician may recommend clearance of athletes for participation. It is often helpful to prepare a list for the coach naming all athletes with a particular problem. For example, a list could name all athletes with tight hamstrings so the coach could instruct them to pay more attention to appropriate stretching exercises.

A preparticipation examination is also extremely useful to recommend matching participants for balanced competition. Low Tanner stage athletes should be in competition with other low Tanner stage athletes. In general, team physicians should recommend against pairing low Tanner stage athletes with athletes in the higher Tanner stages who are more psychologically and physically mature.

If the team physician notes a problem in the examination, she should thoroughly inform the athlete and the athlete's parents about the problem and any specific actions that should be taken to address it. For example, if an athlete has an incompletely rehabilitated anterior cruciate injury, he should be put on a rehabilitation and strengthening program prior to the start of the season.

Besides thoroughly informing the athlete and her parents of any abnormality found in the preparticipation examination, the team physician must recommend whether the athlete should participate. If the athlete or her parents are adamant about participation, the team physician should consider executing an exculpatory waiver accompanied by the highest level of informed consent.

Although athletes who are legally competent may be allowed to sign exculpatory waivers or risk releases, this may not be the case with minor athletes. In many states parents of minor athletes cannot sign exculpatory waivers on behalf of that athlete. Team physicians should contact attorneys familiar with the laws in their states before having parents sign a waiver or allowing athletes to sign for themselves. In many states exculpatory waivers are held to be against public policy, and thus they would not insure that the team physician or the school system could not be sued. In other states, however, exculpatory waivers have been upheld in court.

Athletes who desire to participate against the team physician's recommendations may sue to be allowed to participate under the Federal Rehabilitation Act and the ADA. Athletes who sue under the Federal Rehabilitation Act usually have medical clearance from a physician other than the team physician. In this case, a team physician may allow the athlete to participate against his recommendation if the athlete signs an exculpatory waiver. If the athlete is a minor and desires to participate against the team physician's recommendation or if the athlete resides in a state that invalidates exculpatory waivers, it may be best to allow the athlete to pursue participation through the courtroom. If the court directs the school to allow the athlete to participate and the athlete subsequently suffers a catastrophic injury of the type that the denied clearance was intended to prevent, then it is unlikely that the school system or the physician would be found liable. The ADA has not yet been tested in a sports medicine case.

A Case Citing the Federal Rehabilitation Act

In *Pool v. South Plainfield Board of Education*, the parents of a handicapped child knew the dangers involved in their child's participation in wrestling when he had only one kidney. However, the parents encouraged the athlete's participation. The school district initially excluded the wrestler from participation based on the recommendation of his physician. The federal district court, however, stated that the school district could not deny the student's right to participate. The court said the purpose of Section 504 of the Federal Rehabilitation Act, which makes it unlawful for anyone receiving federal funding to discriminate against otherwise qualified individuals on the basis of a handicap, is to allow handicapped individuals to live life as fully as they are able without authorities determining what is too risky.[36] The court in the Pool case heard testimony from two physicians, a family physician and a doctor from a sports medicine center, that qualified the athlete to participate. The court did not indicate how it would have ruled absent such medical clearance.[37]

References

1. Mellion, M., Walsh, W.M., & Shelton, G.L. (1990). *The team physicians hand book* (p. 19). Philadelphia: Hanley and Beltus.
2. *American Medical Association: Medical evaluation of the athlete: A guide* (rev. ed.) (p. 12). (1976). Chicago: American Medical Association.
3. Goldberg, B., Dyment, P.P., Haefel, S., Murray, J.J., Risser, W.L., & Nelson, M. (1988). Preparticipation sports assessment—an objective evaluation. *Pediatrics*, **66**(736).
4. Durant, R.R., Seymour, C., Linder, C., & Jay, S. (1985). The preparticipation examination of athletes. *American Journal of Diseases of Children*, **139**, 657-663.
5. Runyan, D.K. (1983). The preparticipation examination of the young athlete. *Clin Pediatric*, **22**, 674-677.
6. Smith, N., & Stanitski, N. (1987). *Sports medicine, a practical guide* (p. 4). Philadelphia: W. B. Saunders.
7. Dyment, P. (1992, April 15). The triple threat sports exam. *Journal of Patient Care*, 97-117.
8. McCaffrey. (1991, February). Sudden cardiac death in young athletes. *American Journal of Diseases of Children*, **145**, 177-183.
9. Advice on conditioning is internal to sports physical (1992, April). *Family Practice News*, **22** (7).
10. Kuland, D.K. (1982). *The injured athlete* (p. 27). Lipincott.
11. *Preparticipation physical examination*, a joint publication of the American Academy of Family Physicians, American Academy of Pediatrics, American Orthopedic Society for Sports Medicine, the American Medical Society for Sports Medicine, American Osteopathic Academy of Sports Medicine.
12. Pepper v. City of New Rochelle School District, 531 N.Y.S. 2d 367 (A.D. 2 Dept. 1988).

13. Benitez v. New York, 5300 N.Y.S. 2d 825 (A.D. 1 Rept. 1988).
14. Dyment, P. (1992, April 15). The triple threat sport exam. *Journal of Patient Care*, 97-117.
15. Smith, N., & Stanitski, N. (1987). *Sports medicine, a practical guide* (p. 114). Philadelphia: W.B. Saunders.
16. Cantu, R.C., Micheli, L.J. (Eds.). (1991). *American College of Sports Medicine's guidelines for the team physician* (p. 72). Malvern, PA: Lea & Febiger.
17. PIAA Data Sharing Project, Physician Insurance Association of America, 1985-1991.
18. Thomas & Cantwell. (1990). Case report sudden death during basketball games. *Physicians and Sports Medicine Journal*, **18**(5), 75-102.
19. Siscovic, D.L. (1984). The incidence of primary cardiac arrests during vigorous exercise. *New England Journal of Medicine*, **311**, 874.
20. *British Medical Journal.* (1991, February 2). **302**, 269.
21. Jersaty, R.M. (1986, January). Mitral valve prolapse: Definition and implications in athletes. *Journal of American Cardiology*, **7**(1), 231-236.
22. Herbert, W. G. (1990, June). The death of Hank Gathers: Implications to the standards of care for preparticipation screening. *Sports Medicine Standards and Malpractice Reporter*, **2**(3), 41-46.
23. Herbert, D.L. (1991). The death of Hank Gathers: An examination of the legal issues. *Sports Medicine Standards and Malpractice Reporter*, **3**(6), 45.
24. Maron, B., Roberts, W., McAllister, H., Rosing, D., & Epstein, S. (1980, August). Sudden death in young athletes. *Circulation*, **62**(2), 128-129.
25. Sox, H.C., Garber, A.M., & Littenberg, B. (1989, September). *Annals Int Medicine*, **111**(6), 489-502.
26. Mitchell, J., Maron, B., Epstein, S. (Co-chairs 16th Bethesda Conference). (1985). Cardiovascular abnormalities in the athlete: Recommendations regarding eligibility for competition. *16 Journal of the American College of Cardiology*, **6**, 1183-1232.
27. Georgia House Bill 1711 introduced on 2/17/92.
28. Comodeca, J. (1991). Constitutional rights and participation in interscholastic athletics: The courtroom as the new playing field. *Sports Medicine Standards and Malpractice Reporter*, **3**(3) 47-51.
29. Manno, A. (1991). The high price to compete: The feasibility and effective waivers used to protect schools from liability for injuries to athletes with high medical risks. *Kentucky Law Journal*, **79**, 880.
30. Larkin V. Archdiocese of Cincinnati. Case No. C-1-90-619 (S.D. Ohio 1990).
31. Zappa, J.M. (1991). The Americans With Disabilities Act of 1990: Improving judicial determinations of whether an individual is "substantially limited." *Minnesota Law Review*, **75**, 1303.

32. Grube v. Bethlehem School District, 550 F. Supp. 418 (E.V. Pa. 1982).

33. Lawes, R. (1992, June 1). Larkin gives Longhorns heart to win. *USA Today*, C 1.

34. Herbert, D. (1990, June). The death of Hank Gathers: An examination of the legal issues. *Sports Medicine Standards and Malpractice Reporter*, **2**(3), 45-48.

35. Wichmann, S., & Martin, D.R. (1992, February). Single organ patients. Balancing sports with safety. *Physician and Sports Medicine*, **20**, (2), 176-182.

36. Pool v. South Plainfield Board of Education, 490 F. Supp. 948 (D.C.N.J. 1980).

37. Manno, A. (1991). The high price to compete: The feasibility and effective waivers used to protect schools from liability for injuries to athletes with high medical risks. *Kentucky Law Journal*, **79**, 867-881.

CHAPTER 6

Return-To-Play Decisions

The star quarterback had a history of sustaining "stinger" injuries to his right shoulder and arm but always completely recovered. In the last game of the regular season he again sustained a stinger. By Wednesday the numbness and tingling were still present, although greatly diminished. This was the first time that the athlete did not completely recover almost instantaneously. By Friday morning the numbness was almost but not completely gone. The team physician thought the athlete still experienced tingling, but the athlete denied it. The physician told the coach the athlete could not play in the play-off game the next day. The athlete's parents immediately called the team physician, and the parents and coach tried to persuade her to change her mind and allow the athlete to play. When the team physician did not relent, the parents took the athlete to another physician who pronounced him fit to play.

Questions:

▌ Should the stellar quarterback be returned to play just because he's needed for the play-offs?

▌ How should the team physician handle the pressure from parents?

▌ Is the athlete discounting his symptoms in an effort to be returned sooner than is in his best interests?

▌ Who has the final say in the matter—the coach, the team physician, or an outside physician?

 All these questions may impact the ability of the team physician to fulfill her fundamental obligation to act in the best interest of the athlete.

 Return-to-play decisions are among the most difficult decisions for team physicians. Nowhere are the issues of competing loyalties as clear as when the physician must determine if an athlete can play. This decision is inextricably linked with the issues already considered about the preparticipation exam and the assumption of risk.

Basic Principles

Studies have demonstrated that 65% to 75% of all sports-related injuries occur during practice and training, not during competitive events.[1] Regardless of the situation in which the decision is to be made, team physicians must adhere to return-to-play criteria—contain the pressure to return an athlete to play during competition and adhere to the same criteria they would use if they were evaluating the athlete outside a game situation. The basic principles of return-to-play decisions are clear:

> Before competition, the principle goal of the team physicians is injury prevention; during competition, the primary responsibility is triage of the acutely injured athlete. Post-competition, proper and appropriate rehabilitation is a prime concern.[2]

During competition, the following general guidelines can help team physicians determine whether an athlete can safely reenter or continue to participate:

1. The diagnosis has tentatively or definitively been made.
2. The injury will not be worsened by continued participation.
3. The injury or condition will not place the athlete at increased risk for other injuries or reduce the athlete's capability to protect himself.[2]

One role of the team physician is to minimize out-of-action time. In fact, that is what often sets a good team physician apart form one who is not well schooled in sports and rapid rehabilitation techniques. However, the team physician's duty to keep athletes alive and injury free is an even greater obligation.[3] One of the key goals of the return-to-play decision is avoiding postscreening injury or death.[2] Profiles of specific sports and the specific injuries common in them are widely available, and team physicians should use this information when making the return-to-play decision.[2] For instance, a swimmer who sustains a head injury can be returned to swimming much sooner than a football player with a similar injury can return to playing football because the team physician would be concerned about the second impact syndrome in which an athlete suffers a severe and often fatal injury after sustaining a minor second blow to the head. The goal of these decisions is to allow the athlete to reenter the playing arena as quickly as it is safe to do so.

External Pressures

Team physicians may often feel pulled from different directions—the athlete, the team, and the parents. A team physician's decision regarding returning an athlete to play may be motivated not only by what is in the best interest of the athlete, but also by what is in the best interest of the team and by what the parents demand about the athlete's participation. For example, if a pivotal member of the team is hurt, the athlete's return may be hastened by rapid rehabilitative techniques well known in the literature, the use of special protective equipment, and the motivation of the athlete to adhere to the rehabilitation regimen. These are proper influences on the team physician's decision to return the athlete to play. However, the determination must be made based only on what is in the best medical interest of the athlete and not on what the team, coach, or parents want if their desires are not in accordance with the best interest of the athlete.

In high school athletics, in general, the team physician is not employed by the school system. Remember that employment by the school system, even if only for a nominal fee, can negate the immunity provision of Good Samaritan statutes discussed in chapter 3. Because the team physician is not employed by the school, he owes no duty to the school. Contrast this with the employed college team physician who owes a fiduciary duty to her employer to act in the best interest of the team. The physician's duty to the athlete and the duty to the team and the school can and often do become nebulous. But no such duty exists in the typical relationship between a high school and a team physician. Therefore, a high school team physician is free to legally exercise his judgment determined solely by what is in the best interest of the athlete, unlike the college or professional team physician, whose duty may be clouded.

Consider the example of the star high school quarterback with a grade I concussion. His neurological symptoms, which include only mild postconcussion dizziness, abated within 1 hour. When the team physician evaluates him the Wednesday after the game the athlete is completely asymptomatic with the exception of a mild postconcussion headache. The regional championship games are to begin the next Friday. The quarterback has never been sacked in his 3 years of starting and has never sustained any type of injury on the field—his concussion occurred when he fell off his bicycle. The coach says that the team will protect the quarterback and not allow him to be hit. He points out that there is no back-up quarterback and that without this quarterback the team's chances of winning are nonexistent. Any team physician in these circumstances might be very tempted to return the athlete to participation despite the headache. However, to do so would be inviting disaster, both for the athlete and for the team physician. The reasonably prudent team physician in the same or similar circumstances would be aware of second impact syndrome and would know that athletes with postconcussion headaches should not be allowed to participate in sports in which they are likely to sustain another head injury. If the athlete plays, certainly the team would be happy and well served. But if the athlete gets hit, and there can be no guarantee that he won't, second impact syndrome occurs, and that athlete sustains a severe injury or dies, then the team physician will be defenseless. That the team needed the quarterback is not a defense that will hold up in any courtroom.

This example illustrates the pressures faced by team physicians. Pressure may come from the coach, the team, the parents, or the athletes themselves to return the athlete to play although that decision may not be consistent with sound medical practices under ordinary circumstances.[4] When these pressures come from someone other than the athlete, they must not be allowed to influence the physician's decision regarding care or returning to play. If the coach or other individuals continue to pressure the physician or undermine the physician's decision, then the team physician should document her recommendations and carefully consider terminating her relationship with the team.[4]

A signed contract with the school system that specifies the team physician as the individual who ultimately determines whether an athlete can participate can markedly reduce friction and misunderstanding on this issue.

The Team Physician's Allegiance

Conflicts with the athletes themselves may be more difficult to resolve. Studies have demonstrated that athletes, as a group, significantly underestimate the disruptive effects of injuries.[5] Both athletes who are underage and not legally competent to consent to treatment and athletes who are adults in the eyes of the law can differ with the team physician, with somewhat different consequences.

If an athlete is underage and thus not legally allowed to consent to treatment, don't allow either her or her parents to dictate her care. If the parents insist on pursuing a regimen against the team physician's recommendations, insist that the parents execute an exculpatory waiver. The varied legal interpretations of exculpatory waivers are more fully discussed in chapters 4 and 5. Remember to check state law governing the use of exculpatory waivers for minor athletes.

If the athlete is legally competent to consent to treatment, the matter becomes even more complex and may require considering ethics as well as what the law requires. On the one hand it could be argued that the professional responsibility of the physician transcends even the desires of the patient. Although the team physician's job is to minimize out-of-action time, he has a larger obligation to keep athletes alive and free from further injury.[3] However, others assert that athletes should be managed differently than nonathletes in terms of length of rest and inactivity, since athletes need less rest and cannot withstand inactivity as well as nonathletes.[6] Some argue that the adult athlete should be permitted to accept normally unacceptable risks of participation.[7]

In the past, if there was a risk of significant harm to the athlete, the team physician was almost universally advised not to allow the athlete to participate.[4] In light of the changing legal environment surrounding the use of exculpatory waivers, informed consent, and assumption of risk, that advice has changed. The team physician's recommended course of action now would be to fully inform the athlete of the risks of returning to participation. Next the team physician should advise the athlete not to participate and explain the consequences of her refusal to follow the advice. The physician should then require the athlete to execute an exculpatory waiver before allowing her to return to participation. In those states that do not uphold the use of exculpatory waivers, athletes should not be permitted to play. Athletes may then seek to use the court system to force the issue. Exculpatory waivers are addressed in chapter 4 and preparticipation physician examinations and exclusions from participation are addressed in chapter 5.

Highly Motivated Athletes

Highly motivated athletes commonly want to continue to participate despite medical conditions that make it dangerous for them to do so. Sports medicine is practiced on atypical patients whose decision making is colored by the environment in which they compete.[8] In one example among many, a university football player tried to force the school to allow him to play despite the team physician's decision that he should be benched because of a hyperflexion injury to his neck and the discovery of congenital, cervical spinal stenosis. The player argued that a second doctor's prognosis permitted contact and that benching him would diminish his chances at a pro football career.[9] When the football player was eventually benched, he sued to be allowed to play. The district court refused to hear the suit and thus there has been no ruling. A sample case outlining the difficulties of decision making appears on page 96.

In the case of highly motivated athletes who are legally competent to make their own decisions, the legal concepts of informed consent and assumption of risk guide the team physician's actions. If the athlete is fully informed, this informed consent is documented, and the athlete executes an exculpatory waiver that includes a clause regarding assumption of risk, the team physician will be more likely to avoid liability if the athlete participates against a documented recommendation and then sues.

The Charlie Krueger case illustrates the consequences of a lack of informed consent. Charlie Krueger was the San Francisco 49ers first round draft pick in 1958 and played until 1973. By 1988 he was in constant pain and unable to climb, squat, kneel, lift, stoop, run, jog, or even walk or stand for prolonged periods of time.[10] The court found that in 1963, Krueger was operated on to repair a medial collateral ligament. During the operation, he was found to be anterior cruciate deficient. Krueger was never informed of this or of the consequences of continuing to subject his knees to the rigors of the game. From 1963 until the end of his career he was in chronic pain, was regularly anesthetized between and during games, and underwent repeated steroid injections. Court records document that Krueger was never informed of the deterioration of his knees that was apparent on X rays taken repeatedly over his final playing years. Ultimately the court ordered the 49ers to pay Krueger over $2.3 million in damages, primarily because of the lack of informed consent.[11] The defense argued that Krueger assumed the risk by voluntarily participating in the game of football. However, an athlete cannot assume risk without complete informed consent. In fact, the appellate court in this case found that the 49ers had the requisite intent for a finding of fraudulent concealment, that is, intentionally failing to disclose professionals' warnings to Krueger to which he was clearly entitled.[11]

Involvement of Other Practitioners

Almost every team physician will face a recommendation regarding an athlete's participation from another medical practitioner that is different from his own. Often the discussion with the parents and the coaching staff will end when the team physician reminds them that the contract stipulates the team physician's decisions are final. However, if a team physician receives a recommendation different from her own, it makes sense to reevaluate her recommendation. Perhaps the other decision was based on new research, newer rehabilitative techniques, or new types of protective equipment. Perhaps the other medical practitioner had specialized knowledge of the treatment and consequences of the injury in question. The team physician may want to find out the basis for the other medical practitioner's decision.

If the team physician still stands by his decision after reconsideration, and the parents or the legally emancipated athlete, not the coach, decides to follow the advice of the other medical practitioner, the team physician should follow the process of full informed consent. This includes discussing the risks of returning to participation, explaining that the team physician's recommendation is against participation, and having an exculpatory waiver executed.

New Legal Concerns

Reentry to play decisions may also be affected by the Federal Rehabilitation Act of 1973 and the newly enacted American With Disabilities Act, which were discussed in chapter 5 as they related to exclusions from participation based on the preparticipation examination. The legal concepts are the same, and athletes who have been denied participation may resort to the courts to procure a spot on the team.

When Hank Gathers was allowed to continue to play basketball, the team physician arranged for a defibrillator on the sidelines at all subsequent games.[12] Who should bear the expense for providing specialized equipment or personnel that athletes with health problems require to continue to participate? Although there is no clear legal precedent on the issue, it makes sense that the participant or his family should bear the cost. The athlete will be participating against the team physician's recommendation, so the team physician should not be required to bear the expense. An argument could be made that the team is benefiting from the participation of the athlete and thus should be required to pay. But what if the school system has no discretionary funds for such expenses? In addition, most school systems would probably concur with the recommendations of the team physician, so why should they have to underwrite the cost of providing specialized protective equipment and personnel for possible use of an individual athlete?

The newly enacted Americans With Disabilities Act may affect the issue of who pays for specialized equipment needed by handicapped athletes. The ADA has been interpreted as requiring physicians to underwrite costs incurred to implement the requirements of the ADA. For example, physicians have to underwrite the cost of a sign language interpreter for deaf patients. It can be argued, then, that the ADA may require physicians or the school system to pay for the cost of specialized equipment needed by a handicapped athlete. Because the ADA was only recently implemented, there is no case law or regulations yet on this issue. See page 97 for an example of such a case.

Practical Considerations

The overriding duty of the team physician is always to the athlete. This is true regardless of how much pressure the team physician feels from the coaches, other members of the team, and parents. The team physician is required to give full disclosure to the athlete and the parents regarding the extent of an injury, the nature of the injury, proper rehabilitation, and the consequences of injuries.

The coaches and other members of the administration associated with the team should all be aware that the team physician makes the ultimate determination regarding return-to-play decisions.

If, after full disclosure, the legally competent athlete or the parents, in the case of a minor athlete, insist on contravening the physician's recommendation, the team physician should require an exculpatory waiver. The team physician should fully document his recommendation and the athlete's or parents' choice to forego following the recommendation. The team physician and the school system should seek legal advice from attorney familiar with the laws of the individual state with respect to exculpatory waivers. If exculpatory waivers have been traditionally held to be against public policy in the state, then the team physician should stand firm on her recommendation against participation, the coaches and administration should make it clear that they concur, and the athlete should not be allowed to participate. Without the protection of an exculpatory waiver, the team physician who allows an athlete to participate against her better judgment faces potentially monumental liability.

The athlete or parents may choose to exercise their right of access to the court system and sue for the right to participate. If the court ultimately orders the team physician or the school system to allow the athlete to participate, the liability of the team physician is very low.

If an athlete is allowed to participate, either after the execution of an exculpatory waiver or after a court order, the team physician then has a duty to care for that athlete should a catastrophic injury or disorder occur. That may mean having specialized medical equipment available on the sidelines or making sure that rescue personnel and emergency evacuation equipment are readily available. Who bears the costs for this equipment or personnel should be an item for negotiation when the exculpatory waiver is drawn or when the court deliberates on its order.

The Buoniconti Case

A recent case that highlights the difficulties in athletic decision making is the Nick Buoniconti case. Buoniconti was a linebacker for a college football team. He suffered a series of neck injuries in three consecutive games and was allowed to participate in contact drills during the week prior to a game in which he suffered a paralyzing injury. Subsequently Buoniconti filed a lawsuit against the team doctor who had the responsibility to determine whether Buoniconti could suit up and play in the game.[3]

The major issue at the trial involved the innovative alteration of Buoniconti's helmet. The team physician added a 10-in. fitted strap to Buoniconti's uniform running from the face mask to the shoulder pads.[14] The arguments centered around whether the team doctor was negligent in allowing Buoniconti to play with his history of previous neck injuries and whether the alteration of the equipment by attaching the face mask to the shoulder pads contributed to the injuries or, alternatively, was sufficient protection to allow him to play.[15] The jury found that Buoniconti assumed the full risk of playing and that the doctor was not contributorily negligent. In addition, the jury found that Buoniconti spear tackled—used his head as a spear—which also contributed to his injury.

Although the team doctor was not found to be liable, many questions about the case remain. Was Buoniconti properly instructed about the hazards of spear tackling? Was he properly informed of the increased risk of catastrophic injury that he faced by continuing to participate even with the face mask alteration? Did the alteration make it safer for him to play or did it make it more hazardous?

The Benitez Case

Although not directly on point, a case recently decided in New York may have far-reaching legal effects on the reentry to play decisions of team physicians. Benitez, a high school football player, suffered a broken neck, leaving him paralyzed, during the last few minutes of the first half of a football game played in 1983. His team, over the objections of school authorities, had been promoted to the A division of the football league from the less competitive B division. The school authorities objected to the transfer, citing the poor performance of the team in the prior year in the B division and raising the concern that participation in the more competitive A division could prove to be unsafe. Prior to the game in which Benitez was injured, the coach noted that there was a very high risk of injury and that the game should not be played. Benitez was injured after playing both defense and offense and being on the field virtually the entire game. The evidence disclosed that Benitez was fatigued at the time of his injury, which occurred as he was attempting to clock an opposing lineman. During the trial, Benitez's coach testified that it was unsafe for him to play both offense and defense, and the plaintiff's expert testified that both mismatched competitors and playing while tired increase the risk of injury.

The jury ultimately awarded Benitez $1.2 million, which was subsequently reduced to $825,000. The court concluded that the evidence indicated that the school system unreasonably enhanced or increased the risk of injury by playing Benitez in a game between unmatched teams and by playing him for virtually the entire game, although he was tired, because there was no adequate substitute. The court noted that Benitez never complained of being tired; however, the court maintained that the law recognized a degree of indirect compulsion in student-teacher relationships and that a student may be understandably reluctant to refuse to participate for fear of negative reprisals.[16]

Although the Benitez case was not filed against the team physician it still brings up areas of concern. Many of the ever-increasing practice parameters covering sports medicine practitioners note that team physicians should have the final authority as to who may participate in school programs. After the Benitez decision this may mean that the team physician will be required to remove players like Benitez from the game. But team physicians typically are not involved in coaching. A practical effect of the Benitez decision is that team physicians on the sideline must make a diligent effort to ascertain whether an individual athlete is becoming excessively fatigued. In addition, athletes must be counseled at the beginning of the season and throughout that they *must* voluntarily take themselves out of the game when fatigued.

References

1. Garek. (1977). Sports medicine. *Pediatric Clinics of North America*, **24**, 737-747.
2. McKeag, D.B. (1990, October). Criteria for return to participation. *Sports Medicine Standards and Malpractice Reporter*, **2**(4), 61-69.
3. Fairbanks. (1979, August). Return to sports participation. *Physician and Sports Medicine*, p. 71.
4. King, J.H., Jr. (1981, May). The duty and standards of care for team physicians. *Houston Law Review*, **18**(4), 657-705.
5. Crossman, J., Jamieson, J., & Hume, K. (1990, October). Perceptions of athletic injuries by athletes, coaches, and medical professionals. *Perceptual and Motor Skills*, **71**, 848-850.
6. Shaffer. (1976, December). So you've been asked to be the team physician. *Physician and Sports Medicine*, p. 57.
7. Capron. (1974). Informed consent in catastrophic disease research and treatment. 123 U. Pa. L. Rev. **340**, 364-376.
8. Davis, J. (1988, Fall). Fixing the standard of care: Motivated athletes and medical malpractice. *American Journal of Trial Advocacy*, **12**, 215.
9. Sandefer, G. (1989, February). College athletic injuries: Does the Buoniconti case create a duty of an athlete not to play? *Florida Business Journal*, **63**, 34.

10. Padwe. (1988, June 27). When trust is betrayed. *Sports Illustrated*, p. 80.

11. Krueger v. San Francisco 49ers, 234 Cal. Rptr. 579, 581 (1987) (Cal. App. 1 Dist. 1987).

12. Smith, S. (1900, March 119). The death of a dream. *Sports Illustrated*, **11**.

13. Sandefer, G. (1989, February). College athletic injuries: Does the Buoniconti case create a duty of an athlete not to play? *Florida Business Journal*, **63**, 34.

14. Nack, W. (1988, August). Was justice paralyzed? *Sports Illustrated*, p. 92.

15. Sandefer, G. (1989, February). College athletic injuries: Does the Buoniconti case create a duty of an athlete not to play? *Florida Business Journal*, **62**, 35.

16. Hebert, D., Esq. (1989, July). Reentry to play decisions, new legal concerns. *The Sports Medicine Standards and Malpractice Reporter*, **1**(3), 58.

CHAPTER 7

Legal Aspects
of Equipment Use

At a Friday night midseason football game, a wide receiver sustains a "bell ringer," momentarily blacking out, then gets up and is helped off to the sidelines by his teammates. The team physician examines the athlete and removes him from the game. The athlete's symptoms completely abate and he is returned to the game. On a play in the third quarter he again suffers a concussion.

The player was wearing an old, secondhand helmet that requires players to blow up air bladders to cushion the head. The air bladders in the wide receiver's helmet leaked, and examination of the helmet after the second injury revealed that the bladders were not inflated.

Questions:

▌ Is the team physician liable for the team's choice and use of faulty equipment?

▌ Is the team physical liable if the athlete deliberately deflated the bladders so his helmet would not be so tight?

▌ Does the team physician's liability change because he did not examine the athlete's helmet and ascertain that the bladders were fully inflated after the first event?

Many legal issues surround the prescription and use of equipment by the team physician. What emergency equipment should the team physician have available on the sideline or in the medical bag? How liable is the team physician for equipment choices made by the coach or administration for use by the entire team? What about the liabilities associated with prescribing protective equipment for a particular condition or injury? Legal issues need to be considered when addressing all these questions.

The Medical Bag

In the past, team physicians organized the contents of their medical bags based on what they thought would be needed. Therefore, the contents of the medical bag varied from team physician to team physician. However, the development of the specialized practice of sports medicine has been accompanied by articles and books, many of which contain recommendations for the contents of the team physician's medical bag. These articles may legally affect the team physician, as this scenario illustrates.

A player has an acute emergency on the field that leads to a respiratory arrest. The team physician has no airway in her bag and ventilates the patient with mouth-to-mouth resuscitation. The athlete ultimately survives but with brain damage. Most articles related to the contents of the team physician's bag suggest that it should include an airway. The athlete subsequently sues, maintaining that standard articles in the professional literature state that the team physician should have an E-T tube or airway available and that these articles define the standard of care. The athlete claims that by not having an E-T tube available, the team physician did not meet the standard of care and thus was negligent.

Therefore, it is imperative that team physicians are familiar with the most common recommendations for the contents of the medical bag. Table 7.1 lists contents recommended by the American College of Sports Medicine (ACSM).

It is impractical or even impossible for any one team physician to provide for or carry the entire contents suggested in the ACSM guidelines. The physician may modify the contents of the medical bag for many reasons. If an ambulance is available at every game the team physician would not be required to duplicate the emergency equipment it contains, typically spine boards, sandbags, emergency CPR equipment, drugs, and oxygen. However, the team physician must ascertain beforehand what equipment is actually available in the ambulance, whether the ambulance personnel are trained to use the equipment, and what cardiac life support they can provide. If they are not trained in advanced cardiac life support (ACLS), then they will not have the necessary equipment and drugs on hand for ACLS resuscitation. If ACLS cannot be provided at the scene, it is crucial that the team physician ascertain that the ambulance personnel can quickly transport an injured athlete to an emergency facility. Many of the suggested contents of the medical bag can be kept in the locker room or training room where they are easily accessible during the game and at practice sessions instead of being immediately available on the sidelines. Only the drugs or equipment that would be needed immediately in an emergency must be available of the sidelines.

The contents of the team physician's bag may also be determined by the site of the game. If the game is away, the physician for the home team is

Table 7.1   Recommended Contents of the Medical Bag

Physician's bag

Air cast–type ankle brace	Penlight
Alcohol and povidone-iodine (Betadine) swabs	Prep razor
	Prescription pad
Bandages, including elastic (Ace, Elastoplast), plastic strip (Band Aids)	Prewrap
	Reflex hammer
	Scalpel
Batteries and bulbs (extra)	Scissors
Benzoin	Scrub brushes
Blood pressure cuff	Slings
Cotton swabs	Splints
Eye kit with eye chart	Sterile gloves
Finger splints	Sterile water
Forceps	Steri-strips
Gauze	Stethoscope
Hemostats	Suture kit
Ice	disposable sutures
Irrigation kit	nonabsorbable suture (4-0, 5-0, 6-0)
Measuring tape	
Nasal packing	Syringes and needles
Notepad/Dictaphone	Tape
Otoscope/ophthalmoscope	Thermometer

Field equipment

Air splints	Crutches
Blankets	Sandbags
Bolt cutters	Spine board
Cervical collar (rigid)	Stretcher

CPR equipment

Airway/endotracheal tube	Esophageal obturator
Bulb suction syringe	Intravenous setups (5% dextrose in water and lactated Ringer's solution)
Cardiac monitor/defibrillator*	
Catheters, 14- and 18-gauge	
Crash cart with cardiac and anaphylactic medications	Laryngoscope
	Oral and nasal oxygen with mask

Medications

Analgesics	Antibiotics
Aspirin or acetaminophen	Cephalosporin
Codeine or synthetic analgesic tablets	Erythromycin
	Quinalone (optional)
Morphine sulfate or meperidine injectable	Tetracycline

(continued)

Table 7.1 (*continued*)

Medications (*continued*)	EENT medications
Cardiac medications	Antibiotic ophthalmic drops

Medications (*continued*)

Cardiac medications
  Atropine
  Beta blocker
  Bretylium
  Digoxin
  Dopamine
  Epinephrine
  Furosemide
  Lidocaine
  Nifedipine
  Nitroglycerine
  Sodium bicarbonate
  Verapamil
Dermatologics
  Antibiotic ointment
  Antifungal cream
  Insect repellant
  Silver sulfadiazine cream
  Steroid cream
  Sunscreen
  Sunburn cream
  Zinc oxide powder

EENT medications
  Antibiotic ophthalmic drops
  Pseudoephedrine
  Scopolamine patch
  Tetracaine ophthalmic drops
Gastrointestinal medications
  Antacids
  Antidiarrhetic (Lomotil)
  Antiperistaltic (Loperamide)
  Antispasmodic (Donnatol)
  Bismuth subsalicylate (Pepto-Bismol)
  Prochlorperazine
Miscellaneous
  Albuterol inhaler
  Aminophylline
  Antimalarial/antiparasitic medications
  Clove oil
  Dental packing
  Diazepam, injectable
  Diphenhydramine
  Insulin, regular, human
  Ipecac
  Naloxone
  Xylocaine

Note. From R.C. Cantu & L.J. Micheli: *ACSM's Guidelines for the Team Physician.* Philadelphia: Lea & Febiger, 1991. Used with permission.

*Cardiac monitor/defibrillator, although not mandatory for basic CPR, is required for advanced cardiac life support (usually supplied by the ambulance).

usually responsible for providing emergency resuscitation equipment and drugs. The team physician should ascertain what is available at each of the away game sites.

If a team physician is responsible for an athlete with special health problems, such as Hank Gathers, he is responsible for the immediate availability of emergency equipment the athlete may require whatever the site of the game.

Finally, the team physician must continually update and restock the medications and supplies in his bag. It would be difficult to defend a team physician who used a drug in an emergency situation that did not achieve the desired effect because it had expired.

Prescribing Protective or Rehabilitative Equipment

The team physician frequently must prescribe protective equipment as a prophylaxis against injury, for use during rehabilitation, to allow athletes to return sooner to participation, and as protection after an injury has occurred.

Choosing the Proper Equipment to Prescribe

The first legal issue in the prescription of protective equipment is the choice of the proper piece of equipment. Protective equipment is specialized and, as in all areas of medicine, new devices and applications are being developed constantly. The team physician may face a lawsuit based on an allegation of failure to prescribe the most appropriate piece of protective equipment. Staying clinically competent in the field of sports medicine by attending continuing medical education courses and reading the literature is the best way to avoid being sued over prescribing the wrong piece of equipment.

In addition, allegations that the physician failed to prescribe protective equipment at all may be made. For example, any team physician knows that once an athlete has sustained an ankle sprain, especially a grade II or grade III ankle sprain, she will be more susceptible to repeat ankle sprains.[1] Therefore, the team physician has a duty to ensure that the athlete is properly taped before returning to participation or to prescribe an ankle air cast or some other device to help stabilize the ankle.[2] Failure to prescribe proper taping or a stabilizing brace would be a breach of the duty owed to the athlete, and if the athlete returned to participation and reinjured her ankle, it would be difficult to successfully defend the team physician against a lawsuit. Again, the best way to prevent lawsuits for the failure to prescribe protective equipment is to remain clinically competent in the field.

Ensuring Proper Application of Protective Equipment

Another area of potential liability in sports medicine related to equipment is ensuring that the athlete knows how to properly use special devices. Prescribing a device without demonstrating how to use it is similar to advising a woman to perform breast self-examinations without instructing her in the technique.

If the team physician prescribes an ankle air cast, he should make sure that the athlete knows to wear a heavy sock beneath the air cast, to match his heel to the curvature of the air cast heel, and to properly inflate the air bladders. If the athlete is not properly instructed in all these areas and the air cast is applied improperly, it will not be as effective in preventing a recurrent ankle sprain. The athlete could later claim that if he had been properly instructed in the application of the air cast he would have applied it properly and would not have suffered a recurrent sprain. The same scenario could occur with almost any piece of protective equipment team physicians prescribe. Obviously, the more sophisticated or technical the equipment is, the more likely the athlete will not know how to apply it correctly and the greater the need for the physician to ensure that the athlete has been adequately instructed.

The team physician does not necessarily have to provide the instruction herself, although it remains the physician's duty to be sure the athlete has been adequately instructed. If the team physician works with a trainer, she should develop a routine to inform the trainer when equipment is prescribed to an athlete and to ensure that the athlete is instructed in its use. If the mechanism for instruction is in place and the physician knows that the trainer will adequately instruct the athlete, then she will have met the duty to adequately instruct.

If the athlete fails to follow the instructions after being taught how to use protective equipment properly, it could be argued that the athlete has assumed the risk. If the athlete assumes the risk by not following the proper instructions and subsequently sustains an injury that would have been prevented by using the equipment properly, it would be very difficult to find the team physician liable. By deliberately electing to misapply the equipment the athlete assumed the risk of injury and would probably be unable to shift the burden and liability to the team physician.

Monitoring Protective Equipment Use

If a team physician discovers that athletes are applying equipment improperly, he has the duty of informing the athlete that she is using the equipment inappropriately and ensuring that the athlete is instructed on proper application of the equipment. For example, if an athlete sustains a concussion, the team physician should evaluate whether the bladders in his helmet were properly inflated. If the bladder is improperly inflated, the team physician should instruct the athlete on proper inflation and check the helmet routinely to ensure that the athlete is properly following instructions. The team physician has the duty of continuously monitoring athletes.

Liability for Altered Protective Equipment

One of the major issues in the Buoniconti case discussed in detail in chapter 6 was the issue of the altered helmet. Buoniconti's face mask was attached to his shoulder pads by a strap. This device was used in an attempt to protect him after he withstood several neck injuries, but Buoniconti was paralyzed by a tackle despite the alteration. The court ultimately did not find the team physician negligent in altering the helmet,[3] but the issue was determined on the basis of assumption of risk. The court determined that Buoniconti assumed the risk of further injury when he elected to continue to play despite his recent neck injuries. The case could easily have gone the other way, and the court could have found the team physician liable for the altered equipment because it placed Buoniconti at a higher risk of injury.[4] This case illustrates the potential liability team physicians who alter equipment face. An alteration that may appear to help prevent a certain type of injury may actually place the athlete at a higher risk for a different injury. The team physician should carefully consider all the possible consequences of an alteration before modifying the protective equipment athletes use, and then carefully document why the alteration was made and what he hoped to accomplish by the alteration.

Informed Consent and the Use of Protective Equipment

Protective equipment is designed to protect the athlete from injuries that may be caused by participation. Some equipment, while protecting against certain types of injuries, may also place athletes at increased risk of other injuries. For example, football helmets protect from head injuries, but because they allow the athletes to tackle with their heads, they may place them at increased risk of neck injuries.[5]

Choosing Routine Protective Equipment by Schools

Team physicians are not routinely involved with selecting and maintaining protective equipment such as padding, helmets, shoes, and other equipment designed to prevent injuries that is provided to team members at the start of the season. This equipment is usually chosen by school system coaches and athletic directors. However, as noted in chapter 1 when we discussed practice parameters and standards that govern the practice of sports medicine, a standard set by the American Academy of Pediatrics (AAP) may cause physicians to be potentially liable for the choice of equipment by school personnel.[6]

The AAP states that team physicians are medical advisors to schools in their selection and fitting of equipment.[7]

> One of the most important yet neglected roles of the team physician is the involvement in the choice of protective equipment. Eye, face and head protectors...should be chosen and properly fitted to each athlete. Well made, properly fitted protective devices are as important to beginners as to the more experienced athlete. If used equipment is recycled to the less skilled players, it should be first quality and fit well. There is *no excuse* for having inadequate protective equipment in an athletic program.

> The physician's responsibility for injuries does not start only after an injury occurs. Some coaches tend to minimize the necessity for protective equipment, especially in practice sessions. The authority of the physician in the prevention of injuries must be "spelled out" by the athletic director before the session begins. Even if the team physician has no control over the choice and use of protective equipment, he is vulnerable to legal action when injuries occur which could have been prevented by better designed or better fitting equipment.[7]

Another guideline that may affect the team physician's liability in this area appears in a different AAP publication:

> The team physician should be responsible for assuring that only safe, well fitting, and reliable equipment is used in athletic programs.[8]

The above guidelines obviously place team physicians in potential peril. They suggest that team physicians may have a duty to be involved in assessing, choosing, fitting, and even maintaining all protective equipment used by athletes, not just equipment the physician prescribes.

Plaintiffs' attorneys may maintain that these standards place a duty on the physician to be involved with equipment selection and fitting, which can be especially damaging to team physicians who are pediatricians and belong to the AAP. A plaintiff's attorney could potentially attempt to demonstrate to a jury that physicians should be aware of and follow guidelines promulgated by professional organizations to which they belong. If physicians are not involved in the selection and maintenance of equipment and an athlete is injured because of faulty equipment or ill-fitted equipment, the attorney may argue that the physician was negligent by not following the guidelines.

This is a clear example of how guidelines can place physicians in potential peril. Because team physicians must follow practice guidelines to the best of their ability, it may be judicious for them to become involved in equipment selection and fitting. In some situations, though, it may be highly impractical for them to do so. In other situations, coaches or administrators may not want them involved in equipment selection, fitting, and maintenance. In these cases physicians should consider documenting why it is impractical or impossible to become involved or that they attempted to work with the proper personnel but their attempts were not successful. Chapter 1 provides more in-depth discussion of guidelines and practice parameters.

Even without specific practice parameters, team physicians may have the duty to recommend the use of helmets for participants of certain sports. The effectiveness of bicycle safety helmets in the prevention of head injuries has been widely demonstrated.[9,10] With this information widely available in the sports medicine literature, physicians who counsel cyclists may have the duty to counsel them to use helmets. Once the physician has recommended the use of helmets, if the cyclist then declines to wear the helmet, she can be found to have assumed the risk of riding without adequate protection from head injuries.[11]

Practical Considerations

The team physician is expected to carry a medical bag or ensure the availability of medical equipment on the sidelines. The generally recommended contents of the medical bag can be changed, however, based on the practicality of providing the equipment and the nearby availability of equipment. If an ambulance is on hand, the burden of providing resuscitative equipment may be relieved. In general, the home team physician has the duty to ensure that emergency medical equipment is available on site or very close by.

If the team physician is caring for an athlete with a special need, such as Hank Gathers' need for a defibrillator, she has the duty to provide such equipment. The cost of protective equipment should be discussed before its purchase, but in general it should be borne by the athlete with the special needs. The new Americans With Disabilities Act may modify this guideline in certain situations.

With the team physician's duty to provide emergency resuscitative equipment also comes the duty to know how to provide advanced cardiac life support or to ensure that someone immediately available can provide such resuscitation.

The team physician has the duty to be knowledgeable in prescribing protective equipment, especially injury-specific equipment, whether it is used for prophylaxis, therapy, rehabilitation, or to enable athletes to return to participation more rapidly. To maintain clinical competency in this area, as in any area of medicine, team physicians must continually read the sports medicine literature and attend courses and hands-on workshops.

One of the most neglected areas of equipment use by team physicians is the proper application of protective equipment. Team physicians may know how or why to prescribe a shoulder harness but may not know how to put one on. It is essential that the athlete receive proper instruction regarding the application of protective equipment, and it is the team physician's duty to ensure that this occurs. If the trainer or other individuals are the usual instructors in equipment use, the team physician must develop a process that ensures that no athlete is missed.

If a team physician finds out that an athlete is misapplying equipment, he must ensure that the athlete receives proper instruction, even if the athlete received proper instruction initially. When the team physician is put on notice that misapplication is occurring, he has a duty to rectify the situation at least once. The team physician cannot just ignore the problem. If the athlete continues to misapply the equipment, the doctrine of informed consent may be an issue—it could be argued that by continually misapplying the equipment the athlete assumed the risk of injury. The team physician could also consider requesting that the coach bench the athlete for failing to follow proper instruction.

Team physicians should be wary of altering protective equipment. An alteration that may effectively protect an athlete against one type of injury may place an athlete at an increased risk for another type of injury. If an athlete's injury is caused by the altered equipment, the team physician may potentially face high liability.

The increasingly common development of practice parameters may help protect team physicians but may also potentially increase team physicians' legal perils. Practice guidelines that recommend the involvement of team physicians in the selection, fitting, and maintenance of protective equipment make it advisable that physicians attempt to become involved in these areas or document their efforts if involvement is impractical or impossible. It is essential for team physicians to keep abreast of practice guidelines already in place and practice guidelines being developed.

Because the effectiveness of helmets in protecting against head injury is so well known, the team physician has the duty to advise cyclists to use helmets. Certainly bicycle team physicians should include helmet use in the first discussion with the team and should not allow the participation of athletes who refuse to wear helmets.

References

1. Miller, E., & Hergenroder, A. (1990, October). Prophylactic ankle bracing. *Pediatric Clinics of North America*, **37**(5), 1175-1185.
2. Stover, C. (1980). Air stirrup management of ankle injuries. *American Journal of Sports Medicine*, **8**(5), 360-363.
3. Sandefer, G. (1989, February). College athletic injuries: Does the Buoniconti case create a duty of an athlete not to play? *Florida Business Journal*, **63**, 34.

4. Smith, N., & Stanitski, N. (1987). *Sports medicine, a practical guide* (p. 114). Philadelphia: W.B. Saunders.
5. Ellis, T. (1991, December). Sports protective equipment. *Primary Care,* **18**(4), 889-919.
6. Herbert, D.L. (1990, April). Physician responsibility for provision of safe and effective equipment. *The Sports Medicine Standards and Malpractice Reporter,* **2**(2), 33-35.
7. American Academy of Pediatrics. (1983). *Sports medicine: Health care for young athletes* (p. 4). Elk Grove Village, IL: Author.
8. American Academy of Pediatrics. (1987). *School health: A guide for health professionals* (p. 146). Elk Grove Village, IL: Author.
9. Thompson, et al. (1989). A case control study of the effectiveness of bicycle safety helmets. *New England Journal of Medicine,* **320,** 1361-1367.
10. Sosin. (1989). Head injury—Associated deaths in the United States from 1979-1986. *JAMA,* **262**(16), 2251-2255.
11. Herbert, D.L. (1990, January). Physicians may have duty to recommend helmet use. *Sports Medicine Standards and Malpractice Reporter,* **2**(1), 17.

CHAPTER 8

Potentially Catastrophic Injuries and Conditions

A standout athlete on a local high school basketball team was a known asthmatic. In fact, the team physician had diagnosed the asthmatic condition while performing a routine preparticipation examination. The athlete was well controlled on inhaled medications until one dry winter day when an acute and dramatic exacerbation of her asthma required her to be transported from a game to treatment at a local hospital. Upon investigation it was found that the athlete's inhaler contained medication that was outdated and not appropriate.

Questions:

▉ Now that the team physician is aware that the athlete has a serious asthmatic condition, should he preclude the athlete from playing?

▉ If the athlete continues to participate, what should the team physician do about the athlete's medication? Is the team physician required to keep an emergency supply of bronchodilators available on the sidelines?

▉ What responsibility do the athlete and her family have to keep her medicine refilled appropriately?

Many potential catastrophic injuries can and do occur in sports, but fortunately they are rare—fewer than 1 in 100,000 reported injuries. High school sports produce the highest incidence of injuries in general and also the highest incidence of catastrophic injuries.[1]

A study by the National Center for the Study of Sudden Death in Athletes found that of 118 explained deaths in a 3-year period, 53 were due to cardiac causes, 41 involved trauma such as head injury, 10 were due to heat stroke, 8 were caused by asthma, and 6 were due to cardiac trauma.[2] Because catastrophic injuries can result in significant impairment or death, they often result in lawsuits. To avoid liability, team physicians should be able to recognize what type of situations can lead to catastrophic injuries or life-threatening situations, institute methods of prevention, and know how to properly manage such injuries or conditions should they occur.

Head Injuries

Head injuries occur often in sports. The leading cause of death from head injuries is intracranial hemorrhage.[1] Up to 20% of high school football players suffer concussions in a single season.[3] If an athlete is unconscious it is not difficult to recognize that a head injury has occurred and proper management can be instituted. However, the athlete who receives a "ding" to the head may represent a diagnostic and management dilemma.

Second Impact Syndrome

Athletes with symptoms of a concussion that did not cause a loss of consciousness are at risk for potentially fatal rapid brain swelling and herniation after a second impact to the head,[4] the recently identified second impact syndrome. Between 1980 and 1991, 29 cases of probable second impact syndrome were identified in football players alone.[5] The team physician should recognize the syndrome because prevention is primary. Second impact syndrome occurs when an athlete sustains an initial head injury, anything from a mild concussion to a cerebral contusion. The athlete returns to competition before the symptoms of the previous injury resolve and sustains a second blow, which may be minor, to either the head or the body. The second blow transmits accelerative forces to the brain. The athlete may appear to be stunned but usually remains conscious. Within a few seconds to several minutes the athlete collapses and becomes semicomatose. The athlete's pupils dilate rapidly, eye movement is lost, and eventually respiratory failure occurs.[5]

The team physician must be able to recognize that the syndrome has occurred and institute treatment on the field. More importantly, the team physician must recognize that second impact syndrome can be prevented by not allowing athletes who have sustained a head injury to return to participation until all symptoms related to the head injury have completely resolved, even symptoms of mild headache, no matter how long they persist.[5]

Team physicians should be familiar with the diagnosis and treatment of other potentially catastrophic head injuries including subdural and epidural hematomas, intracranial hemorrhage, and delayed brain injury.[1]

Neck and Spinal Injuries

Head and neck injuries cause the most football-related deaths.[6] Sports account for about 14.2% of back injuries. The act of diving (not the sport of diving) accounts for about 66% of sports-related back injuries; football, 6.1%; wrestling, 2.3%; and gymnastics, 2.2%.[7]

Spearing in football, which is blocking or tackling head first, is a major cause of paralyzing injuries. Spearing is illegal in both college and high school football. Since spearing was outlawed, the number of paralyzing injuries has fallen precipitously. Nevertheless between 1977 and 1989 there still were 122 paralyzing injuries at the high school and junior high football levels.

A case dating back to 1958 underscores the importance of properly moving an athlete who may have sustained cervical spine trauma. In *Welch v. Dunsmuir Joint Union High School District*, Welch, a high school football player, was tackled after he took the ball on a quarterback sneak. As he was falling forward, another player coming in to make the tackle fell on top of him. Welch was unable to get up. The coach suspected a neck injury and attempted to elicit grip strength from Welch; there was none. The evidence is in conflict as to whether the team physician directed the subsequent move of Welch by eight fellow athletes or whether the move was undirected. Nevertheless, the trial court found that moving Welch without the use of a stretcher was an improper medical practice and subject to liability.[6]

The team physician's responsibility in the face of a neck or spinal injury centers around appropriate management. The most important management criteria is how to move an athlete with a suspected neck or spinal cord injury. Team physicians should be well acquainted with techniques for moving an injured athlete that will insure that the cervical spine is stabilized. One of the most common mistakes made by team physicians, coaches, and fellow athletes is to remove football players' helmets when they have sustained a neck injury. If the athlete has sustained a neck injury, removing the helmet can be potentially devastating, rendering a paralyzing injury to the athlete from an unstable cervical vertebral fracture. The team physician or other personnel should never remove the helmet on the field if a neck injury is suspected, even if the athlete is unconscious. If the athlete's airway needs to be cleared, remove the face mask rather than the helmet.[2] This axiom is fairly well known. It is not hard to envision the liability a team physician may face if a player goes down on the field and can move his limbs and then the football helmet is removed and the player becomes paralyzed. Refer to page 117 for an example involving a life-threatening condition of an athlete.

Cardiovascular-Induced Sudden Death

Among athletes under the age of 35, the most common cardiac etiology of sudden death is congenital heart disease.[9] A recent study of athletes who died suddenly revealed that hypertrophic cardiomyopathy is the most common structural anomaly, followed by idiopathic left ventricular hypertrophy.[10] The most important method of preventing sudden death is to detect athletes at risk during the preparticipation exam. Intensive screening results in a very low yield. Using a screening questionnaire that specifically asks the athlete about a family history of premature death, a history of steroid or cocaine use, and other conditions and diagnoses associated with cardiac abnormalities can help identify at-risk athletes and markedly decrease the team physician's liability.[10] In addition, the 16th Bethesda Conference of the American College of Cardiology developed specific recommendations regarding the eligibility for competition of athletes with cardiovascular abnormalities. The incidence of cardiovascular-induced sudden death in athletes with identified cardiovascular abnormalities can be reduced by following these recommendations.[11]

Acute Respiratory Emergencies

Several acute respiratory emergencies can affect athletes, including exercise-induced bronchospasm, exercise-induced anaphylaxis, cholinergic urticaria, and seasonal allergic problems.[12] Athletes susceptible to any of these respiratory conditions can usually be detected with a screening questionnaire that specifically asks the athlete about these conditions. Team physicians should be thoroughly familiar with respiratory conditions and have pharmacologic support on hand or nearby so they can begin treatment rapidly and effectively.

Heat Illness

Heat illnesses range from benign heat cramps to heat exhaustion to potentially fatal heat stroke. The most important precept regarding heat illnesses is that they are all preventable.[13] Identify athletes at risk for heat injury during the preparticipation examination. During high heat and humidity, restrict their athletic activity and increase their water intake.[14] Some team physicians use a sling psychrometer, which measures the levels of heat and humidity, or other devices to determine the level of danger.[2] Restrict players who lose 3% or more of their body weight during a workout from activity until rehydrated.[14] Develop and implement general heat policies. Finally, recognize the development of heat illness in athletes and remove the athlete experiencing symptoms from the game. Heat stroke is a life-threatening emergency that demands immediate intervention. Be prepared to provide immediate resuscitative treatment.[14]

A tragic case of the heat stroke death of an athlete demonstrates the necessity of recognizing heat illnesses when they occur and properly managing them. A high school football player suffered heat stress during a practice session. The athlete was sent to the locker room without a proper evaluation or examination. In the locker room the athlete became unconscious, but no medical evaluation or treatment commenced until approximately 1 hour and 20 min later. The athlete died and his parents sued the school board, contending that the coach failed to perform the duty of providing all necessary and reasonable safeguards to prevent accidents, injuries, and sickness of the football players. The parents ultimately won the lawsuit.[15]

Practical Considerations

Catastrophic injuries can cause significant physical impairment or death. Potential legal damages are high, which often prompts the injured athlete or his family to sue, and they may name the team physician in the lawsuit. The most important defense against a suit is for the team physician to recognize the potential for catastrophic injury, institute preventive programs, and appropriately manage the situation should it arise.

The most common catastrophic injuries are head injuries, cardiac conditions, acute respiratory emergencies, and heat illness. Athletes susceptible to these conditions can usually be identified by using a screening questionnaire during the preparticipation examination. Team physicians should have proper resuscitative equipment immediately available for use if the situation demands it.

The Tragic Story of Reggie Lewis

Reggie Lewis was a 27-year-old Boston Celtics professional basketball team standout and team captain. During the first half of the first game of the NBA playoffs he collapsed. He was brought to the sidelines and examined and returned to play in the second half only to collapse again. Lewis was hospitalized and a team of seven cardiologists examined him and determined he suffered from hypertrophic cardiomyopathy, the same affliction that killed Hank

Gathers. He was told his basketball career was over, and his team physician concurred. Lewis checked himself out of that hospital and into another one where a different cardiologist examined him. This cardiologist came up with an altogether different diagnosis than the first team did. He stated that he found that Lewis had neurogenic cardiovascular syndrome—a condition that causes the heart rate to slow down when exercise should cause it to accelerate. The cardiologist noted that the condition was treatable with medication and that Lewis could return to his basketball career. He then developed a program of monitoring Lewis while Lewis was doing treadmill exercises in preparation for basketball season.

A few weeks after the cardiologist's statement, Lewis was shooting baskets before participating in a pick-up game of basketball, collapsed, and died. An autopsy revealed that the first diagnosis, that of hypertrophic cardiomyopathy, was correct. After Lewis died it came to light that he was seeking the advice of a third physician or set of physicians, indicating that he still had some concerns over the recommendation that he could play.

Among the questions that arise from this case are these:

Who has precedence—the team physician or an outside physician who was sought out by Lewis (who after all was an adult who could make his own decision regarding his multimillion-dollar career)?

Was Lewis adhering to the regimen requiring monitoring while exercising?

Lewis was not exerting himself strenuously while shooting the baskets. Therefore, regardless of the conflicting diagnoses, Lewis was at high risk of dying with the least bit of exertion, the type of exertion that occurs in everyday life. Therefore, if Lewis had followed the recommendations there is no assurance that he would not have collapsed while carrying out everyday activities.

References

1. Cantu, R.C., & Micheli, L. (Eds.) (1991). *ACSM's guidelines for the team physician* (pp. 143-150). Philadelphia: Lea & Febiger.
2. Results of a three-year study of sudden death in athletes. (1992, September 15). *Family Practice News*, **22**(18), 17.
3. Blake, J. (1991, December 12). Head injury without blackout may still be fatal. *Medical Tribune*, **32**(25).

4. Kelley, J., Nichols, J., et al. (1991). Concussion in sports: Guidelines for the prevention of catastrophic outcomes. *JAMA*, **226**(20), 2867-2869.

5. Cantu, R. (1992, September). Second impact syndrome. *Physician and Sports Medicine*, **20**(9), 55-66.

6. Statement by Fred Mueller, M.D., head of the National Center for Catastrophic Sports Injury Research at the University of North Carolina.

7. Robert, T. (1991, November 2). Lineman for Lions paralyzed by injury. *New York Times*, B9 (national edition).

8. Welch v. Dunsmuir Joint Union High School District, 326 P. 2d 633 (Cal. App. 1958).

9. Andes, P. (1992, September). Preventing sudden death. *Physician and Sports Medicine*, **29**(9), 75-89.

10. Epstein, S., & Maron, B. (1986). Sudden death and the competitive athlete: Perspectives on preparticipation screening studies. *Journal of the American College of Cardiology*, **7**(1), 220-230.

11. Mitchell, J., Maron, B., & Epstein, S. (Co-chairs, 16th Bethesda Conference). (1985). Cardiovascular abnormalities in the athlete: Recommendations regarding eligibility for competition. *16 Journal of the American College of Cardiology*, **6**, 1183-1282.

12. Adelman, D., & Spector, S. (1989, January). Acute respiratory emergencies in emergency treatment of the injured athlete. *Clinics in Sports Medicine*, **8**(1), 71-78.

13. Murphy, R. (1992, September 1). Statement at the first annual meeting of the American Medical Society for Sports Medicine as quoted in *Family Practice News*, **22** (17).

14. Mellion, M., Walsh, W., & Shelton, G. (1990). *The team physicians handbook* (pp. 59-69). St. Louis: Hanley and Belfus Inc. Mosby-Yearbooks.

15. Mogabgab v. Orleans Parish School Board, 239 So. 2d 456 (Court of Appeals, La. 1970).

CHAPTER 9

Athlete Drug Use

A track star wants to improve his sprinting times and has heard in the locker room that steroids will help him build more muscle and more muscle will help him improve his time. He starts taking steroids to increase his bulk, which they do. He soon wants to quit using steroids both because he knows that he will be tested and because he doesn't feel right about using them. He asks the team physician about the safest way to wean himself of the steroids. The team physician gives him appropriate advice and gradually the athlete becomes steroid free. Prior to participating in Olympic trials he catches an upper respiratory infection and asks the team physician for something to help him feel better. The physician tells him to take an over-the-counter decongestant. He does, feels better, and wins a spot on the Olympic team. When he is drug tested he is found positive for sympathomimetics and is removed from the team. His sponsor, a major shoe company, releases him from his contract as a spokesman for their product.

Questions:

▌ Does the team physician face liability because of advising the athlete about the appropriate and safe way to discontinue using the steroids?

▌ Should the team physician inform the proper authority about the athlete's steroid use?

▌ Is the team physician liable for the athlete's use of an over-the-counter banned substance?

▌ Is the team physician liable for the athlete's loss of income as a result of being released from the spokesperson contract?

Drug use is pervasive in our society and prevalent among athletes. A survey by Heitzinger and Associates found that from 1981 through 1986 90% of high school athletes had used alcohol; 45%, marijuana; 21.5%, amphetamines; and 17%, cocaine. A recent study in Texas found that 6.7% of male high school athletes used anabolic steroids.[1] Another study found the rate of anabolic steroid use in male athletes as high as 11%.[2] Growth hormone has now become a frequently abused drug in athletics, and the statistics suggest that its abuse rate is at or near the abuse rate found for anabolic steroids.[3] Many athletes who use anabolic steroids also use human growth hormones.[4] The team physician can play a pivotal role in preventing drug abuse in athletes.

Why Athletes Use Drugs

Many physicians and drug counselors contend that athletes use drugs because they believe that drugs will enhance their athletic performances.[5] Usage is the result of the pressure to win, to have an edge over the competition, or to keep up with the competition that the athletes believe are using drugs to enhance their performance. Some athletes believe they need drugs to "get up" before competition or to "come down" after competition.[6]

Commonly Abused Drugs

Drugs can be separated into three different categories: therapeutic, performance enhancing, and mood altering. Therapeutic drugs, or drugs prescribed by a physician to treat a medical problem or injury, are not addressed in this chapter. Alcohol, marijuana, and cocaine are mood-altering drugs, and anabolic steroids and human growth hormone are performance-enhancing drugs.

Alcohol

The most commonly abused drug is alcohol. Athletes may use alcohol for its calming effect, to escape from reality, or because of peer pressure. The detrimental effects of alcohol are well known. A statement by the American College of Sports Medicine explains how alcohol use relates to athletic performance:

1. The acute ingestion of alcohol has a deleterious effect on many psychomotor skills, including reaction times, hand-eye coordination, accuracy, balance, and complex coordination.

2. Alcohol consumption does not substantially influence physiologic functions crucial to physical performance ($\dot{V}O_2$max, respiratory dynamics, cardiac function).

3. Alcohol ingestion will not improve muscular work capacity and may decrease performance levels.

4. Alcohol may impair temperature regulation during prolonged exercise in a cold environment.[7]

Marijuana

Marijuana use is still quite prevalent—according to one estimate 17 million Americans regularly use the drug.[8] Many athletes who use marijuana first try the drug while in high school or junior high school.[9] Marijuana, like alcohol, is used primarily for its euphoric effect. The adverse effects of marijuana use include a reduction of maximal exercise performance, with premature achievement of $\dot{V}O_2$max and inhibition of sweating, which can lead to an increase in core body temperature.[10,11] Marijuana also can cause tachycardia, an increase in systolic blood pressure while supine and decreased standing blood pressure, impaired motor coordination, decreased short-term memory, difficulty concentrating, and a decline in work performance.[11] Finally, marijuana also causes decreased plasma testosterone, gynecomastia, and oligospermia.[12]

Cocaine

Cocaine is another mood-altering drug, although occasionally it is used by athletes as an ergogenic aid because it acts as a central nervous system stimulant.[13] Athletes also may use cocaine to improve performance by masking or helping to postpone the onset of fatigue. Its use is so common, according to a 1987 New York Times article, that "Cocaine has probably joined rotator-cuff injuries, torn ligaments, and broken bones as a potential occupational hazard for athletes."[14] Cocaine has many deleterious and potentially life-threatening side effects, including ventricular dysrhythmia, coronary vasospasm with thrombosis, and myocardial infarctions, all in patients without underlying heart disease.[15] In addition, cocaine use has been found to result in agitation, insomnia, tremulousness, toxic psychosis, severe depression, paranoia, and dysphoria.[15] Cocaine has direct effects on the ability of the brain to regulate body temperature, causing an athlete exercising in the heat to be susceptible to hyperthermia.[16] Athletes who abuse cocaine often use the drug with individuals other than teammates, perhaps making it more difficult for team physician to detect its use.

If a whole team or parts of a team are abusing cocaine, the physician may be able to discern a pattern, thus enabling detection of abusers.[9,17]

Anabolic Steroids

About one third of high school users of anabolic steroids begin using the drug before the age of 15.[18] The main reasons they cite for using anabolic steroids are to improve performance, for appearance, to prevent or treat a sports injury, and for social reasons.[9] Anabolic steroids increase muscle size and strength when the person taking them is performing strenuous strength training and is on a diet that includes sufficient protein.[19] Steroid use can cause hepatocellular dysfunction and poliosis hepatitis and it can increase the chance of the athlete developing hepatocellular carcinoma.[20] Anabolic steroid use can also increase low density lipoprotein (LDL) and total cholesterol and decrease high density lipoprotein (HDL), elevate blood pressure, and possibly cause myocardial infarction and cerebrovascular accidents.[21] Anabolic steroids often cause psychological effects including changes in libido, mood swings, and aggressive behaviors.[22] Anabolic steroid use can produce oligospermia, decreased testicular size, and gynecomastia in males and can cause reduced leutenizing hormone (LH)/follicle stimulating hormone (FSH), estrogens, and progesterone; menstrual irregularities; male pattern baldness; hirsutism; cliteromegaly; and deepening of the voice in females.[21] The changes that occur in the female athlete are often irreversible. Anabolic steroid use among youths may cause irreversible, premature closing of the epiphysis.[22] This is ominous in light of the frequency of anabolic steroid use in youths aged 15 or younger.

Human Growth Hormone

Human growth hormone use is on the rise among athletes. There is controversy and debate in the medical and scientific literature about whether growth hormone increases muscular strength, but it does increase muscular growth,[23] which is undoubtedly why athletes use human growth hormone. The most potentially serious side effect of athletes abusing human growth hormone, especially those abusing megadoses, is the development of acromegaly, which can lead to diabetes, arthritis, and myopathies.[23] The facial bones may become coarse because of the overgrowth of the brow, the jaw, and other soft tissues, and the heart, lungs, and liver may double in size.[24]

Drug Sources

Alcohol is freely available to athletes, who either purchase it directly or receive it from friends and family. Illicit drugs, such as cocaine, marijuana, and amphetamines, are available "on the streets." Athletes obtain anabolic steroids from a variety of sources in a vast, multifaceted black market made up of a heterogeneous mix of coaches, veterinarians, athletic trainers, pharmaceutical industry employees, and others.[25] The black market contributes as much as 80% of the steroids used by American athletes and is reported to gross as much as $200 to $400 million per year.

Another source of anabolic steroids is physicians. Physicians prescribe steroids for a variety of reasons including a misguided but genuine belief that it is in the best interest of the athlete. Other physicians prescribe steroids for monetary gain, and still others may prescribe to satisfy a desire to be affiliated with a sports team or a superstar.[26]

In 1990 the Anabolic Steroid Control Act was enacted. This act puts steroids in Schedule III, the same class as barbiturates and codeine combinations. Possession of these substances without a prescription is a federal offense subject to 1 year in prison and a minimum $1,000 fine. Any physician who prescribes anabolic steroids for other than legitimate purposes could be sentenced to 5 years in prison and fined up to $250,000 under the act. However, it is widely believed that instituting a federal prohibition on illegitimate drug use will not solve the problem of steroid abuse among high school athletes.

Steroids: Team Physician Roles and Responsibilities

A recent survey in Texas revealed that 55% of family physicians surveyed reported being asked about steroids or seeing possible steroid users in their practices. High school boys were the subject of 60% of the inquiries, 26% of which came from parents and specifically pertained to athletes. Football and athletics in general were the most common reasons for inquiry.[27] This study illustrates the opportunity that physicians have to discuss the use of drugs with athlete abusers and their parents.

Athletes may approach the team physician for a steroid prescription directly. Obviously the answer should be a firm no, but don't lose the opportunity to discuss the use of steroids or other drugs for performance enhancement.

Athletes frequently attempt to enlist the team physician's help in monitoring their health while on the steroids. Although this may present a moral or ethical dilemma for a physician, again the opportunity for discussion should not be lost.

Finally, athletes may seek the advice of a physician when discontinuing steroid and other drug use. Again, this is an opportune time to discuss the use of the drug in detail.

Many team physicians refuse to monitor athletes while they are on steroids or refuse to counsel them about discontinuing steroid use.

However, monitoring steroid use in patients who want to continue using these drugs may allow the physician to develop a relationship with the athlete that will give him the opportunity to help the athlete stop using anabolic steroids. It is not illegal to give advice about how to alleviate some of the harmful effects of steroid use, just as physicians and other health care providers provide information to IV drug users about how to avoid becoming infected with the HIV virus. The team physician should be careful not to give the athlete the impression that she condones the use of steroids or other performance-enhancing drugs and should make it clear that the opposite is true. This information should be documented in the athlete's record.

The American College of Sports Medicine, the American Academy of Pediatrics, the International Olympic Committee on Drugs, and the American Osteopathic Academy of Sports Medicine have all developed recommendations that condemn the use of anabolic steroids and urge physicians to ask patients about steroid use during preparticipation physical examinations.

Often physicians wonder what kind of information to give to athletes about anabolic steroids, growth hormone, and their effect. Physicians are much more effective in changing attitudes about steroid abuse if they give balanced information about the potential benefits as well as the risks of using anabolic agents.[27] Providing information only about the adverse effects of anabolic steroid use is unlikely to be effective.[28] These conclusions can be extrapolated to provide information about growth hormone. In fact, it may be advisable to discuss both anabolic steroids and growth hormone at the same time.

Confidentiality

Athletes will not seek help or advice from a team physician whom they cannot trust to keep their confidence—regardless of whether they want advice about performance-enhancing drugs or other, less sensitive matters. With the enactment of the Anabolic Steroid Control Act of 1990, athletes may be reluctant to disclose their drug use to physicians for fear that they will be turned over to authorities. However, the confidentiality of the physician-patient relationship allows the physician to assure athletes that disclosures, discussions, and treatments will remain confidential.

Physicians, however, may have a duty to warn third parties of impending harm related to an athlete's drug use, and a team physician's public duty to warn may override the private duty of confidentiality. Anabolic steroids are known to cause personality changes and heighten aggressiveness and may cause law-abiding and psychiatrically asymptomatic individuals to develop manic and psychotic symptoms culminating occasionally in violent crimes.[30] Physicians must consider properly reporting patients developing these tendencies. This duty was illustrated in a 1990 case in which a physician prescribed steroids to a police officer who was trying to get in shape for the police olympics. The officer developed a steroid-induced psychosis, became violent, and shot three individuals. The court held that the physician had overmedicated the patient with anabolic steroids and testosterone to the point that he became a toxic psychotic. The court held that it was possible to foresee that the officer was likely to attack the victim, and thus the doctor had a duty to warn the victim that she was in danger of physical harm.[29]

Team physicians will, more likely than not, rarely care for athletes who tell them they are going to "get" someone. Certainly, if an athlete is on anabolic steroids and has exhibited a heightened state of aggressiveness and admitted to the physician that he has violent feelings toward someone, that physician may have a duty to warn the possible victim. But in reality, the athlete usually exhibits more aggressive behavior than usual (which is a tip-off that the athlete is abusing steroids) without becoming or threatening to become overly violent. In this case the team physician's duty of confidentiality to the athlete is paramount.

Drug Testing

Drug testing in professional and collegiate sports has occurred for many years, and it is gradually moving into the high school athletics arena. The alarming increase in illegal drug use in schools has forced educators to pursue policies that were virtually unheard of a few years ago. As a result school systems are turning to extensive educational programs and to drug testing to combat the influx of drugs into the school environment. Students and schools are battling in the courtroom over students' constitutional rights such as the right to privacy in relation to drug abuse prevention programs.[31]

Team physicians may be called on to develop, oversee, or participate in drug testing programs. These requests can place the team physician in a difficult situation. If team physicians are involved in selecting athletes for testing, it is doubtful the athletes would trust them and come to them about their drug usage, no matter how often the physician reassured them that such discussions would not be used as a basis for selection for drug testing. Further, involvement in testing and reporting may place team physicians in a precarious legal position. An athlete might sue the team physician for breach of the patient-physician confidential relationship.[32] In addition, physicians who test and monitor for drug programs frequently receive remuneration, which may preclude coverage under any applicable Good Samaritan statute.

However, as drug testing has become more common, more experts recommend that team physicians *do* participate as medical review officers because team drug programs have been viewed as supportive of the athlete and helpful rather than punitive. Team physicians probably should volunteer to work with the school in setting up the drug testing system and developing guidelines for what athletes to test if they have knowledge or expertise in the area or are willing to procure the information.[32] However, if a physician is necessary for testing and reporting aspects of the program and he will be paid for these services, the physician must consider the effect his participation may have on his role as a team physician, as an unbiased and available confidant.

Team physicians are also obvious participants in the educational and counseling portions of drug abuse prevention programs. Again, this is an opportunity for the team physician to have an open, frank, honest, and balanced discussion with athletes who have tested positive for drugs. The confidential physician-patient relationship extends to such educational and counseling sessions, even if the athlete is required to attend them. The confidential nature of the discussion can help engender trust.

Substance Abuse Policies and Guidelines

Athletic organizations, both amateur and professional, have restricted drug use in an effort to maintain a degree of competitive fairness.[33] The two major governing bodies for amateur athletics in the United States are the U.S. Olympic Committee (USOC) and the National Collegiate Athletic Association (NCAA).

The USOC is a member of the International Olympic Committee (IOC), which has developed a list of banned drugs (see Table 9.1).

The major rationale for the IOC's drug banning is to discourage drug use to improve training or performance.[33] Its program is solely designed to guarantee fair competition in amateur sports; the IOC does not classify recreational or street drugs.[33]

The USOC conducts drug testing, using several methods of urine testing.[34] Physicians who also serve as team physicians cannot conduct the drug-control program. Athletes are disqualified if they test positive or refuse to be tested. If an athlete withdraws from a competition because of formal testing, no penalty is imposed.[35]

The NCAA compiled its list of banned drugs similar to the IOC list in 1986 (see Table 9.2). The NCAA also includes substances banned for specific sports, diuretics, and street drugs, but it does not include narcotic analgesics, which are on the IOC list.[33] The NCAA conducts drug testing at 73 championships and football postseason bowl games. Athletes with the most playing time are tested at these events as well as a random sampling of athletes with infrequent playing time.[33]

Table 9.1   Drugs banned by the International Olympic Committee, 1985-1988[a]

Psychomotor stimulants	Narcotic analgesics
Amphetamine	Anileridine
Benzphetamine	Codeine
Chlorphentermine	Dextromoramide
Cocaine	Dihydrocodeine
Diethylpropion	Dipipanone
Dimethylamphetamine	Ethylmorphine
Ethylamphetamine	Heroin
Fencamfamin	Hydrocodone
Meclofenoxate	Hydromorphone
Methylamphetamine	Levorphanol
Methylphenidate	Methadone
Norpseudoephedrine	Morphine
Pemoline	Oxycodone
Phendimetrazine	Oxymorphone
Phenmetrazine	Pentazocine
Phentermine	Pethidine
Sympathomimetic amines	Phenazocine
	Thebacon
Clorprenaline	Trimeperidine
Ephedrine	
Etafedrine	**Anabolic steroids**
Isoetharine	Clostebol
Isoproterenol	Danazol
Methoxyphenamine	Dehydrochlormethyltestosterone
Methylephedrine	Fluoxymesterone
Miscellaneous central	Mesterolone
nervous system stimulants	Methandienone
	Methenolone
Amiphenazole	Methyltestosterone
Bemegride	Nandrolone
Caffeine[b]	Norethandrolone
Doxapram	Oxandrolone
Ethamivan	Oxymesterone
Leptazol	Oxymetholone
Nikethamide	Stanozolol
Picrotoxin	Testosterone[c]
Strychnine	

[a]Information provided by the U.S. Olympic Committee.
[b]If urine concentration exceeds 15 _g/mL.
[c]If ratio of total urine concentration of testosterone to epitestosterone exceeds 6. Based on information in Wagner, J.C. (1987). Substance-abuse policies and guidelines in amateur and professional athletics. *American Journal of Hospital Pharmacy*, **44**, 305-310.

Table 9.2   Drugs banned by the National Collegiate Athletic Association, 1986[a]

Psychomotor stimulants

Amphetamine
Benzphetamine
Chlorphentermine
Cocaine
Diethylpropion
Dimethylamphetamine
Ethylamphetamine
Fencamfamin
Meclofenoxate
Methylamphetamine
Methylphenidate
Norpseudoephedrine
Pemoline
Phendimetrazine
Phenmetrazine
Phentermine
Pipradol
Prolintane

Sympathomimetic amines

Clorprenaline
Ephedrine
Etafedrine
Isoetharine
Isoprenaline
Methoxyphenamine
Methylephedrine
Phenylpropanolamine

Miscellaneous central nervous system stimulants

Amiphenazole
Bemegride
Caffeine[b]
Crolethamide
Cropropamide
Doxapram
Ethamivan
Leptazol
Nikethamide
Picrotoxin
Strychnine

Anabolic steroids

Clostebol
Dehydrochlormethyltestosterone
Fluoxymesterone
Mesterolone
Methandienone
Methenolone
Nandrolone
Norethandrolone
Oxandrolone
Oxymesterone
Oxymetholone
Stanozolol
Testosterone[c]

Substances banned only for riflery

Atenolol
Alcohol
Metoprolol
Nadolol
Pindolol
Propranolol
Timolol

Diuretics

Bendroflumethiazide
Benzthiazide
Bumetanide
Chlorothalidone
Cyclothiazide
Ethacrynic acid
Flumethiazide urosemide
Hydrochlorothiazide
Hydroflumethiazide
Methyclothiazide
Metolazone
Polythiazide
Quinethazone
Spironolactone
Triamterene
Trichlormethiazide

(continued)

Table 9.2 (*continued*)

Street drugs
Amphetamine
Cocaine
Heroin
Marijuana[d]
Methamphetamine
THC (tetrahydrocannabinol)

[a]Information provided by the National Collegiate Athletic Association.
[b]If urine concentration exceeds 15 _g/mL.
[c]If ratio of total concentration of testosterone to that of epitestosterone in the urine exceeds 6.
[d]Based on a repeat test.
Based on information in Wagner, J.C. (1987). Substance-abuse policies and guidelines in amateur and professional athletics. *American Journal of Hospital Pharmacy*, **44**, 305-310.

A student athlete who tests positive (in accordance with the testing methods authorized by the Executive Committee) shall remain ineligible for all regular-season and postseason competition during the time period ending one calendar year after the student athlete's positive drug test, and until the student athlete retests negative (in accordance with the testing methods authorized by the Executive Committee) and the student athlete's eligibility is restored by the Eligibility Committee. If the student athlete tests positive for the use of any drug, other than a "street drug" as defined in 31.2.3.1, after being restored to eligibility, he or she shall lose all remaining regular-season and postseason eligibility in all sports. If the student athlete tests positive for the use of a "street drug" after being restored to eligibility, he or she shall be charged with the loss of one season of competition in all sports and also shall remain ineligible for regular-season and postseason competition at least through the next calendar year.[36]

Professional sports have lagged behind the NCAA and other amateur sports in drug testing, partially because of lobbying by players associations and unions on the right to privacy and civil liberty.[33] The National Basketball Association (NBA) and National Football League (NFL), however, do have programs in place.

The NBA and the NBA Players Association instituted an antidrug program in 1983. In this program an independent expert may issue an authorization which allows the NBA to administer drug tests. The testing procedure consists of four tests, for cocaine and heroin only, in a 6-week period without prior knowledge of the player. The antidrug program provides that any player who is convicted of or pleads guilty to a crime involving the use or distribution of heroin or cocaine, or who is found through the procedure outlined in the agreement to have illegally used these drugs, will immediately be dismissed from the league. The player may seek reinstatement after 2 years. Players may come forward voluntarily to seek treatment of a drug use problem. The treatment program is paid for by the NBA club and the player continues to receive full salary during it. If a player submits a second voluntary request for treatment, he receives treatment but is no longer eligible to receive full pay. Any subsequent illegal use of drugs, even if voluntarily disclosed, results in immediate permanent dismissal from the NBA.

The NFL's comprehensive drug testing policy involves testing all players in the preseason or when they report. In addition, players are subject to reasonable cause testing as medically determined, in-season and off-season. Players who test positive or who are involved in drug-related misconduct are required to obtain a substance abuse evaluation to assess the extent and effects of any chemical dependency and to help formulate a treatment plan.

With the first positive test the player receives notice, evaluation, and treatment as directed by a physician advisor to the NFL. A second positive test results in the removal of the player from the active roster for six games without pay. The third positive test results in the player being banned from further NFL play for at least 1 year. The player then may petition the commissioner for reinstatement.

Team physicians should be aware of the substances banned by amateur athletes, including the International Olympic Committee and the NCAA, and substances that the Professional Sports League tests for and bans. If a team physician inadvertently prescribes a banned substance to an athlete, its use can jeopardize the athlete's career. The athlete could then allege that the team physician negligently prescribed the medication and sue the team physician for damages.

Practical Considerations

Almost every high school team physician has or will have contact with an athlete who is using drugs. The athlete may be abusing legal drugs, such as alcohol or caffeine, or using illegal drugs to enhance performance. The team physician should remember that alcohol is an illegal drug for most high school athletes because they are underage. High school students are increasingly using anabolic steroids and growth hormone as muscle building aids. As many as 90% of high school students have used alcohol, 5.5% to 12% have used anabolic steroids, and 5% have used growth hormone.

The team physician should be thoroughly familiar with the most common signs of drug use, including an abrupt or gradual change in motivation and other behavioral changes such as increased aggression, and should watch for them. If signs are present, the team physician should discuss drug use with the athlete in private, assuring the athlete that the discussion will be kept in the strictest confidence.

The team physician should be thoroughly familiar with not only the risks of the most commonly abused drugs, but also the benefits. The team physician should acknowledge that drugs such as growth hormone and anabolic steroids do in fact increase muscle mass. A balanced discussion helps athletes realize that the team physician is providing information, not preaching. They will be more receptive to learning about the risks and using that information to make a choice about drug use.

The team physician generally does not have a duty to report an athlete who voluntarily discloses drug use to the coach or any other authority. Such a disclosure may potentially place the team physician in a precarious legal position. The team physician should welcome the athlete who wants to discuss his drug use and use the opportunity to discuss the benefits and risks of using the drug. Such a discussion can also occur during the preparticipation sports examination, depending on how much time is available. Some team physicians also present information regarding drug use at the initial team meeting. This is also an opportunity for the team physician to inform the athletes that she is available for *confidential* discussions regarding the use of performance-enhancing drugs and the use of drugs in general.

References

1. Windsor, R., & Dimitru, D. (1989, October). Prevalence of anabolic steroid use by male and female adolescents. *Medicine and Science in Sports and Exercise*, **21**(10), 494-497.
2. Johnson, M.D., Jay, M.S., Shoup, B., & Rickert, V.I. (1989). Anabolic steroid use by male adolescents. *Pediatrics*, **83**, 921-924.
3. Growth hormone abuse may be a new problem in teenage athletes. (1992, July 1). *Family Practice News*, **22**(13), 18.
4. Elias, M. (1982, March 19). Growth hormone use cited. *USA Today*.
5. Sports and drug abuse. (1984). Senate Hearings 98-1220 before the Subcommittee of Alcoholism and Drug Abuse of the Senate Committee on Labor and Human Resources, 98th Congress, 2d Sess.
6. Rose, L., & Girard, T. (1988, Spring). Drug testing in college and professional sports. *University of Kansas Law Review*, **36**(3), 785-821.
7. American College of Sports Medicine. (1982). Position statement on the use of alcohol in sports. *Medicine and Science in Sports and Exercise*, **14**, 9-10.

8. Powell, D. (1987, October). Does marijuana smoke cause lung cancer? *Primary Care and Cancer*, p. 15.

9. Anderson, W.A., & MacKeag, D.B. (1985, June). The substance abuse habit of college student athletes. Mission, KS: National Collegiate Athletic Association.

10. Renaud, A.M., & Cormier, Y. (1986, June). Acute effects of marijuana smoking on maximal exercise performance. *Medicine and Science in Sports and Exercise*, **18**(6), 685-689.

11. Gilman, A.G., Goodman, L.S., Rall, T.W., & Murad, F. (Eds.) (1985). *Goodman and Gilman's the pharmacological basis of therapeutics* (7th ed.) (pp. 1440-1458). New York: MacMillan.

12. Biron, S., & Wells, J. (1983). Marijuana and its effects on the athlete. *Athletic Training*, **18**, 295-303.

13. Puffer, J.C., & Green, G.A. (1990). In M. Mellion, W.M. Walsh, & G.L. Shelton (Eds.), *The Team Physician's Handbook* (pp. 111-127). Philadelphia: Hanley Beltus.

14. Goodwin, M. (1987, May 3). In sport, cocaine's here to stay. *New York Times*.

15. Cregler, L.M. (1986). Special report: Medical complications of cocaine abuse. *New England Journal of Medicine*, **315**, 1495-1500.

16. Giammarco, R. A. (1987). The athlete, cocaine, and lactic acidosis: A hypothesis. *American Journal of Medical Science*, **294**, 412-414.

17. Adelman, D., & Spector, S. (1989, January). Acute respiratory emergencies in emergency treatment of the injured athlete. *Clinics in Sports Medicine*, **8**(1), 71-78.

18. Buckley, W.E., et al. (1988, December 16). Estimated prevalence of anabolic steroid use among male high school seniors. *JAMA*, **260**(23), 3441-3445.

19. Strauss, R. (1991). Chapter 29 drug use and abuse. In Canty, R., & Micheli, L. (Eds.), *American College of Sports Medicine's guidelines for the team physician* (pp. 287-296). Malvern, PA: Lea & Febiger.

20. Overly, W.L., Dankoff, J. A., Wang, B.K., & Singh, U. D. (1984, January). Androgens and hepatocellular carcinoma in an athlete. *Annals of Internal Medicine*, **100**(1), 158.

21. Frankle, M.A. (1989, November). Anabolic androgenic steroids and a stroke in an athlete: Case report. *The Journal of Muscular Skeletal Medicine*, pp. 69-88.

22. American College of Sports Medicine. (1987). Stand on the use of anabolic-androgenic steroids in sports. *Medicine and Science in Sports and Exercise*, **19**(5), 534-539.

23. Macintyre, J.G. (1987, March-April). Growth hormone and athletes. *Sports Medicine*, **4**, 129-142.

24. Strauss, R.H., Wright, H.E., Finderman, A.M., & Catlin, D.H. (1983). Side effects of anabolic steroids in weight trained men. *Physician and Sports Medicine*, **11**(12), 87-96.
25. Bidwell, M., & Katz, D. (1989). Injecting new life into an old defense: Anabolic steroid induced psychosis as a paradigm of involuntary intoxication. *University of Miami Entertainment and Sports Law Review*, **1**, pp. 26-101.
26. Murphy, P. (1986, June). Steroids, not just for athletes anymore. *Physician and Sports Medicine*, **14**, 48.
27. Salva, P., & Bacon, G. (1991, May). Anabolic steroids: Interest among parents and nonathletes. *Southern Medical Journal*, **84**(5), 552-556.
28. Goldberg, L., Bents, R., Bosworth, E., et al. (1991, March). Anabolic steroid education and adolescents. *Pediatrics*, **87**, 283.
29. Webb v. Jarvis, 533 N.E.2d, 151 Ind. APP. 1 Dist. 1990.
30. Pope, H.G., & Katz, D.L. (1990, January). Homicide and near homicide by anabolic steroid users. *Journal of Clinical Psychiatry*, **51**(1), 28-31.
31. Scott, M. (1989, Spring). Is innocence forever gone? Drug testing high school athletes. *Missouri Law Review*, **54**(2), 425-442.
32. Herbert, D.L. (1990). *Legal aspects of sports medicine*. Canton, OH: Professional Reports.
33. Wagner, J.C. (1987, February). Substance abuse policies and guidelines in amateur and professional athletics. *American Journal of Hospital Pharmacy*, **44**(2), 305-310.
34. Drug testing in sports: A round table. (1985). *Physician and Sports Medicine*, **13**, 69-82.
35. United States Olympic Committee. (1985, July). *USOC drug control program protocol, 1985-8*. Colorado Springs: Author.
36. National Collegiate Athletic Association. (1992, July). *NCAA drug-testing/education programs*. Mission, KS: Author.

CHAPTER 10

AIDS, the Athlete, and the Team Physician

A high school wrestler has a history of using intravenous (IV) drugs. In the off-season he is hospitalized for the surgical treatment of a fracture sustained in an auto accident. During that hospitalization he was tested for the HIV virus because needle marks were noted and was found to be positive. He wants to continue to wrestle, and the next fall he tries out and makes the wrestling team. During one of his wrestling matches he sustains a minor laceration to his lip that bleeds. He brushes off any attempt to halt the match and stop the bleeding, noting that he has had these cuts before and they always stop on their own.

Questions:

▌ Should the team physician allow the wrestler to participate?

▌ If the team physician knows that the wrestler is HIV positive, should the coach, team members, and opponents be informed?

▌ What is the appropriate method of handling the bleeding laceration?

AIDS has been present as a diagnosed disease since the early 1980s. The World Health Organization estimates that 8 million people worldwide were infected with HIV at the end of 1990 and predicts that the total will be 40 million by the year 2000.[1] With the high incidence of HIV, high school, college, and professional athletes will be affected.

The stunning disclosure by Ervin "Magic" Johnson in 1991 that he tested HIV positive, his subsequent retirement, reentry, and re-retirement has focused the sporting world on HIV in the athletic arena. Team physicians should be acquainted with the nature of the HIV virus; its mode of transmission; guidelines developed by various organizations regarding

HIV, AIDS, and athletes; and state and organizational requirements for mandatory HIV testing.

Transmission of the HIV Virus in Athletics

To date transmission of the HIV virus by sports contact is suspected in only one documented case. In Italy, a 25-year old man collided with an HIV-positive player during a soccer match. The contact caused both men to sustain severe eyebrow lacerations that bled copiously. One month after the injury the 25-year-old developed symptoms of mononucleosis and 2 months after the injury, he was found to be HIV positive. One year prior to the injury he had been tested and found to be HIV negative. The man denied use of IV drugs, homosexuality, blood transfusions, injections, travel to Africa, and dental care and had been in a stable monogamous heterosexual relationship.[2] Many questions remain about whether this case does indeed represent sports transmission of the HIV virus.

The risk of infection from skin exposure to blood-borne substances from an athlete infected with HIV is unknown. However, studies of health care workers have demonstrated that of 27 confirmed cases of occupationally acquired HIV disease, 7 were a consequence of infected blood splashed onto mucous membranes or the skin.[3] Some authorities believe that an HIV-infected athlete with an unprotected bleeding wound poses a real risk to other competitors if the infected blood comes into contact with or is rubbed into an open skin lesion.[4] Others believe that a more plausible route of transmission is the indirect transfer of blood by a damp sponge or similar first aid equipment used on both players' wounds.[5]

In a 1991 statement, the Committee on Sports Medicine of the American Academy of Pediatrics noted that the risk of infection from skin exposure is minute and is less than the risk of HIV infection by needlesticks from infected patients by a ratio of approximately one case from skin exposure to every 250 cases from needlesticks.[6] The statement further asserts that the report of sports transmission of the HIV virus from Italy remains undocumented.

Potentially High-Risk Sports

The Olympic Committee's policy on HIV transmission, developed by a group of team physicians, notes that the chances of transmitting the virus during sports are extremely low, but that participants in three sports would be at greater risk than others. These three sports are tae kwon do, boxing, and wrestling. The Committee listed basketball as a moderate risk sport.[7] The American Academy of Pediatrics statement suggests that HIV-positive athletes participating in sports involving potential blood exposure such as wrestling and football should be strongly encouraged to consider participation in another sport.[6] Thus it seems that the sports that generate the most concern about the possible transmission of the HIV virus through contact are wrestling, boxing, tae kwon do, and football. These activities obviously carry with them a high rate of injuries in which bleeding occurs, and the bleeding may be accompanied by close bodily contact.

Excluding Athletes From Participation

Currently no regulations require athletes infected with the HIV virus to be excluded from sports. Athletes infected with the HIV virus, more likely than not, would be deemed to be handicapped under the Federal Rehabilitation Act of 1973. This act is more fully discussed in chapter 5. Although no case of an athlete excluded from play because of HIV has reached the courts, *School Board of Nassau County v. Airline*, a case about a person suffering from tuberculosis, determined that tuberculosis did render the person handicapped.[8] Therefore, it can be anticipated that if an athlete is excluded from participation, she may sue under the Federal Rehabilitation Act to be allowed to participate in sports. In addition, the recently enacted Americans With Disabilities Act also specifically notes that AIDS is a handicap. Thus, it is likely that it will apply to HIV-infected athletes who want to participate in contact sports.

Ray v. School District of DeSoto County determined that an AIDS-infected student could not be excluded from classroom enrollment, attendance, and related activities and educational services and opportunities but could, however, be excluded from contact sports.[9] Thus, it appears that some courts may be willing to restrict participation in certain sports activities. In addition, the U.S. Department of Education has stated that medical considerations may justify a school district placing limitations on specific activities by a child infected with AIDS, and such activities may include sports.[10] However, the court determination and the U.S. Department of Education's recommendation must be viewed in light of the Federal Rehabilitation Act of 1973 and the recently enacted Americans With Disabilities Act. It is likely that athletes who are excluded from contact sports, especially the high-risk sports, will sue to be allowed to participate. As this case law evolves, team physicians will be better able to determine what the law requires them to do about excluding athletes from participation in potentially high-risk sports.

Regulations Relating to HIV and Sports

The National Basketball Association (NBA) currently provides a long-term program of disease prevention education and information to all 27 NBA teams. These include the common sense precaution of removing and bandaging a bleeding athlete. The NBA recommendations are based on the World Health Organization Consensus Statement—Consultation on AIDS and Sports. See pages 141-142 for the WHO guidelines on HIV.

At a 1992 meeting, the NBA circulated its recommendations to the National Football League, National Hockey League, major league baseball, the National Collegiate Athletic Association, and the National Federation of State High School Associations. Although the NFL and NCAA have adopted their own specific guidelines, the other groups seemed to agree to follow the recommendations.[11]

The NCAA had already adopted guidelines developed by the Occupational Safety and Health Administration (OSHA). The NCAA guidelines provide that whenever an athlete suffers a laceration or wound that oozes or bleeds, the practice or game must be stopped and the athlete removed from activity for appropriate treatment.[12]

Mandatory Testing for HIV

In 1988 the State of Nevada became the first state to announce mandatory HIV testing for athletes in boxing.[13] However, Nevada's law seems to be an isolated occurrence; no other such recommendations regarding mandatory testing have been made. The NCAA has noted that mandatory testing should not be considered as an alternative to a sound educational program that emphasizes prevention.[11] Team physicians should check with attorneys familiar with the laws in their states to ascertain whether the law mandates testing athletes. This issue is controversial, and the law is evolving.

Practical Considerations

The field of law related to HIV infection and AIDS is changing. The most common lawsuits in this area so far have been related to HIV status and confidentiality and failure to diagnose. Team physicians should take great care to thoroughly familiarize themselves with the World Health Organization guidelines on HIV and the guidelines developed by the American Academy of Pediatrics and to follow them. Both of these guidelines relate to participation of HIV-infected athletes, care for them, and the confidentiality of information about them. The Magic Johnson saga has raised the consciousness of America regarding HIV and athletes. Team physicians are in a prime position to properly educate parents, athletes, coaches, administrators, and the general public about AIDS and athletes and to dispel misinformation.

The WHO Guidelines on HIV

The World Health Organization, with contributions from the American College of Sports Medicine, has developed a consensus statement that reads as follows:

The consultation developed the following consensus statement:

1. No evidence exists of a risk of transmission of the human immunodeficiency virus (HIV) when infected persons engaging in sports have no bleeding wounds or other skin lesions. There is no documented instance of HIV infection acquired through participation in sports. However, there is a possible very low risk of HIV transmission when one athlete who is infected has a bleeding wound or a skin lesion with exudate and another athlete has a skin lesion or exposed mucous membranae that could possibly serve as a portal of entry for the virus.

2. The possible very low risk of HIV transmission through sports participation would principally involve the combative sports with direct body contact and other sports where bleeding may be expected to occur. In such sports, the following procedures should be considered:
   a. If a skin lesion is observed, it should be immediately cleansed with a suitable antiseptic and securely covered.
   b. If a bleeding wound occurs, the individual's participation should be interrupted until the bleeding has been stopped and the wound is both cleansed with an antiseptic and securely covered or occluded.

3. As in other health care settings, for the safety of personnel drawing blood samples from athletes, protective gloves should be worn.

4. Sports organizations, sports clubs and sports groups have special opportunities for additional meaningful AIDS education of athletes, sports officials and ancillary personnel.
   The following should constitute the core of information provided:
   a. HIV can be transmitted through sexual intercourse, blood, and from infected mother to child. Sexual transmission can be either man to woman, woman to man, or man to man, and transmission by blood can include any injection practice in which nonsterile needles and/or syringes are used.

    b. For transmission of HIV through blood to occur during sport, the blood of an infected person must contaminate a lesion/wound or mucous membrane of another person. It should be the responsibility of any athlete participating in a combative sport with direct body contact who has a wound or other skin lesion to report it immediately to a responsible official, and to report for medical attention.

    c. HIV is not transmitted through saliva, sweat, tears, urine, respiratory droplets, handshaking, swimming, pool water, communal bath water, toilets, food or drinking water.

5. There is no medical or public health justification for testing or screening for HIV infection prior to participation in sports activities.

6. Persons who knew they are HIV infected should seek medical counseling about further participation in sports in order to assess risks to their own health as well as the theoretically possible risk of transmission of HIV to others.

7. Sports organizations, sports clubs and sports groups should be aware of the above recommendations and ensure that all participants, sports officials and ancillary personnel are aware of them. In addition, this may provide the opportunity for reviewing general hygienic practices relating to sports.

8. National level sports organizations are urged to contact national acquired immunodeficiency syndrome committees or programmes for further information regarding HIV infection and acquired immunodeficiency syndrome (AIDS).[14]

Note. From the *Consensus Statement From Consultation on AIDS and Sports* by the World Health Organization and the International Federation of Sports Medicine, 1989. Copyright 1989 by the World Health Organization. Reprinted by permission.

The American Academy of Pediatrics Guidelines

The American Academy of Pediatrics Committee on Sports Medicine and Fitness developed a statement regarding HIV in an effort to answer these questions: Should an athlete known to be infected with HIV be allowed to participate in competitive sports and should the universal precautions recommended for health care workers be used when handling athletes' blood and body fluids? These recommendations are as follows:

The American Academy of Pediatrics recommends:

1. Athletes infected with HIV should be allowed to participate in all competitive sports. This advice must be consid-

ered if transmission of HIV is found to occur in the sports setting.

2. A physician counseling a known HIV-infected athlete in a sport involving blood exposure, such as wrestling or football, should inform him of the theoretical risk of contagion to others and strongly encourage him to consider another sport.

3. The physician should respect an HIV-infected athlete's right to confidentiality. This includes not disclosing the patient's status of infection to the participants or the staff of athletic programs.

4. All athletes should be made aware that the athletic program is operating under the policies in Recommendations 1 and 3.

5. Routine testing of athletes for HIV infection is not indicated.

6. The following precautions should be adopted:

   a. Skin exposed to blood or other body fluids visibly contaminated with blood should be cleaned as promptly as is practical, preferably with soap and warm water. Skin antiseptics (e.g., alcohol) or moist towelettes may be used if soap and water are not available.

   b. Even though good hand-washing is an adequate precaution, water-impervious gloves (latex, vinyl, etc.) should be available for staff to use if desired when handling blood or other body fluids visibly contaminated with blood. Gloves should be worn by individuals with nonintact skin. Hands should be washed after glove removal.

   c. If blood or other body fluids visibly contaminated with blood are present on a surface, the object should be cleaned with fresh household bleach solution made for immediate use as follows: 1 part bleach in 100 parts of water, or 1 tablespoon bleach to 1 quart water (hereafter called "fresh bleach solution"). For example, athletic equipment (e.g., wrestling mats) visibly contaminated with blood should be wiped clean with fresh bleach solution and allowed to dry before reusing.

   d. Emergency care should not be delayed because gloves or other protective equipment are not available.

   e. If the care giver wishes to wear gloves and none are readily available, a bulky towel may be used to cover the wound until an off-the-field location is reached where gloves can be used during more definitive treatment.

    f. Each coach and athletic trainer should receive training in first aid and emergency care and be provided with the necessary supplies to treat open wounds.

    g. For those sports with direct body contact and other sports where bleeding may be expected to occur:

        1. If a skin lesion is observed, it should be cleansed immediately with a suitable antiseptic and covered securely.

        2. If a bleeding wound occurs, the individual's participation should be interrupted until the bleeding has been stopped and the wound is both cleansed with antiseptic and covered securely or occluded.

    h. Saliva does not transmit HIV. However, because of potential fear on the part of those providing cardiopulmonary resuscitation, breathing (Ambu) bags and oral airways for use during cardiopulmonary resuscitation should be available in athletic settings for those who prefer not to give mouth-to-mouth resuscitation.

    i. Coaches and athletic trainers should receive training in prevention of HIV transmission in the athletic setting; they should then help implement the recommendations suggested above."[15]

Note. Reproduced by permission of *Pediatrics*, Vol. 88, page 640. Copyright 1991.

References

1. Goldsmith, M. (1991, November 12). Global full-court press against HIV, AIDS spurred by players infection. Medical News and Perspectives. *JAMA*, **266**(20).

2. Torre, D., Sampoetrp, C., Ferraro, G., & Zeroli, C. (1909, May 4). Transmission of HIV-1 infection via sports injury letter. *Lancet*, **335**, 1105.

3. Ciesielski, C.A., Bell, D.M., Chamberland, M.E., et al. (1990). When a houseofficer gets AIDS. *New England Journal of Medicine*, **332**, 1156.

4. Loveday, C. (1990, June 30). HIV and sport (letter). *Lancet*, **336**, 1532.

5. Hoffman, P., & Cookson, B. (1990, June 23). HIV disease and sport (letter). *Lancet*, **336**, 1532.

6. American Academy of Pediatrics Committee on Sports Medicine. (1991, September). Statement, human immunodeficiency virus in the athletic setting. *Pediatrics*, **88**(3), 640-641.

7. Goldsmith, M. (1992, March 11). When sports and HIV share the bill, smart money goes on common sense. Medical News and Perspectives. *JAMA*, **267**(10), 1311-1314.

8. School Board of Nassau County v. Airline, 107 S. Ct. 1123 (1987).

9. Ray v. The School District of DeSoto County, Case Number 87-88-CIV-FPM-17(c) (M) Md. Florida, August 5, 1987.

10. U.S. Department of Education. (1988, January). *AIDS and the education of our children: A guide for parents and teachers* (3rd printing) (p. 19). Washington, DC: U.S. Department of Education.

11. Goldsmith, M. (1991, November 12). Global full-court press against HIV, AIDS spurred by player's infection. Medical News and Perspectives. *JAMA*, **266**(20), 1312.

12. National Collegiate Athletic Association. (1993). *NCAA sports median handbook*, Overland Park, KS: Author.

13. Gunby, P. (1988, March 18). Boxing: AIDS? Medical News and Perspectives. *JAMA*, **259**(112), 1613.

14. World Health Organization in collaboration with the International Federation of Sports Medicine. *Consensus Statement for Consultation on AIDS and Sports*. (1989, January 16). Geneva, Switzerland: Author.

15. Human immunodeficiency virus [acquired immunodeficiency syndrome (AIDS) virus] in the athletic setting. (1991, September). *Pediatrics*, **88**(3), 640-641.

CHAPTER 11

The Physician-Client Relationship

A family physician is employed by the local college to act as a team physician. The physician receives a very small sum of money for his efforts. During a hockey game, the highest scoring athlete in the college's history sustains a severe knee strain. The team physician suspects an anterior cruciate tear, probably a grade III. After the game the team physician receives a call from the local paper. The reporter inquires about the athlete's ability to return to play that season. The team physician tells the reporter that the athlete will never be able to participate in sports again.

The reporter calls his friend, a professional hockey scout, who then decides not to pursue the athlete to discuss a professional career. The athlete recovers completely after surgery and extensive rehabilitation but professional teams are no longer interested in having him join their ranks.

Questions:

▮ Is the team physician an employee of the college or would the team physician be considered an independent contractor? What difference does it make?

▮ Was it appropriate for the team physician to disclose information about the athlete's condition to the press?

▮ How much information should the team physician disclose to the college about the athlete's condition?

▮ Is the team physician liable to the athlete for his loss of potential future earnings?

The collegiate or professional team physician is distinct from the high school team physician in selection, hiring, and remuneration. Team physicians in the professional arena may have more autonomy than those associated with high school and other amateur sports. These parameters have an effect on the legal relationship between the team physician, the athlete, and the hiring entity.

Employee or Independent Contractor

One of the first issues the collegiate or professional team physician must address is whether he is viewed legally as an employee of the university or professional team or as an independent contractor. The distinction is important because it determines whether the university or professional team can be liable for the actions of the team physician.[1] This may be a less important consideration for the team physician than for the entity that hires him because of the doctrine of *vicarious liability*. This doctrine imposes liability on an entity that was not personally negligent, but is held liable because of its relationship with the individual who committed a tort.[2] A tort is a civil, as opposed to a criminal, wrong.

In the sports medicine arena, the most typical relationship that gives rise to vicarious liability is the employer-employee relationship when the team employs the physician. This vicarious liability situation is also described as the doctrine of *respondeat superior*, which is a Latin term for "look to the higher man up."[2] Vicarious liability imposes liability for a negligent act committed by the team physician on the university or team management because of the legal relationship between the physician and the university or team.

Paying a team physician does not automatically make the university or professional sports team liable for her actions. The liability of the employer hinges upon the degree of control the employer exercises over the team physician and how much discretion the team physician has in making decisions.

If an individual is hired by an entity, yet works with little supervision and makes decisions independently of the employer's influence, that person is usually viewed as an independent contractor and is liable for his own negligent acts, not the employer. An independent contractor is a person who, although connected to the employer, is not under the employer's control. Thus if an individual is determined to be an independent contractor, no vicarious liability is imposed. Because collegiate or professional team physicians usually practice autonomously, although they are employed by a university or professional team they are generally held to be independent contractors, not employees, for liability purposes. Again the key determining factor is whether the hiring entity exercises control over the independent judgment of the team physician.[2] As an independent contractor, if the team physician is found to be liable the liability is not imputed to the university or professional team.[2]

In the case of *Cramer v. Hoffman*, a university football player participated in a football game within a few days of his discharge from the hospital where he had been treated for German measles. During the game he sustained severe cervical injuries, which he alleged were a consequence of the negligence of the team physician in moving and treating him. The team physician was found to be negligent but his negligence was not imputed to the school system. The court held that an institution is not responsible for the negligence of physicians who are independent contractors exercising their own discretion and that no evidence introduced proved any type of agency relationship between the team physician and the university.[1]

As in this case, courts generally look to the degree of control exercised by the employee's supervisor over the actual medical decisions. If physicians exercise independent judgment and control they are not employees or agents but rather independent contractors.[2]

Some courts have found otherwise, but these cases are unusual. In *Chuy v. Philadelphia Eagles Football Club*, the team physicians made false statements about Chuy to the press. The court found that the Eagles football club had the right to control and actually did control the substance of the team physician's statements to the press concerning the physical conditions of the athlete. The court noted that the club had no direct control over the team physician's surgical duty and for those purposes the team physician was an independent contractor, but his activities as a spokesman were as an agent of the football club. Thus the club was vicariously liable for the team physician's actions.[3]

Workers' Compensation

An athlete employed by a professional sports team is subject to workers' compensation laws.[2] Workers' compensation laws are not uniform; they vary markedly from state to state. In general, workers' compensation laws limit the amount athletes can recover for their injuries and for negligent acts of their employers. Workers' compensation laws preclude workers from suing their employers for negligence. Therefore, a team physician who commits a negligent act may be protected from a lawsuit if the court determines he is an employee. The following case illustrates the effect workers' compensation laws may have on limiting injured athletes' recovery of damages.

In *Ellis v. Rocky Mountain Empire Sports, Inc.*, Ellis, a former professional football player, sued his team, head coach, team physician, and orthopedic clinic, alleging that he was required to engage in contact football drills before he had fully recovered from an off-season injury. Ellis injured his knee playing basketball during the off-season. One month later he was traded to the Denver Broncos, underwent knee surgery, and began a rehabilitation program under the direction of the Bronco organization. Subsequently he was injured in a contact drill and missed an entire season, ultimately failing a physical and being put on waivers. Ellis alleged that the Broncos required him to engage in football drills before he had fully recovered, that this activity caused further damage to his knee, and that he was entitled to compensatory damages. The district court and the court of appeals ruled that Ellis's sole remedy was in workers' compensation and that he could not sue the club and the team physician employed by the club. Ellis sought to avoid this result by contending that the Broncos organization had intentionally committed the negligent acts of inflicting emotional distress and outrageous conduct and that intentional torts were not covered by the Workers' Compensation Act. The court held that intentional torts are covered under the act.[4]

Good Samaritan Statutes

As discussed in chapter 3, high school and other voluntary team physicians may be protected from lawsuits filed against them for negligence by Good Samaritan statutes. These are state laws enacted to promote voluntarily helping an individual in need. The Good Samaritan doctrine, as a matter of law, precludes negligence liability for a person who sees and attempts to aid another person who has been placed in peril.[2] Good Samaritan statutes generally protect only those team physicians who receive no remuneration for their activities as team physicians. Many collegiate and professional team physicians receive compensation, so they cannot rely on Good Samaritan statutes for protection for acts that may be interpreted as negligence. The receipt of remuneration essentially takes away the measure of protection afforded by the Good Samaritan statutes.

The Doctor-Patient Relationship

If the team physician is to have a duty to act in a certain manner toward athletes who are patients, he must have an established physician-patient relationship with the athlete. The team physician's allegiance to the physician-patient relationship with the athlete is paramount. However, when a physician works for a university or professional team the relationship can become somewhat more complicated. When the team physician is hired by a university or a professional sports team a duty is created not only to the athlete but also to the hiring entity. These "dual duties" begin with the preparticipation examination.

The Preparticipation Examination

As discussed in chapter 5, the primary purpose of the preparticipation examination is to determine the fitness of the athlete to participate. The team physician clearly owes a duty of care to the athlete whether or not the team physician or athlete is employed by the university or professional team.

Notwithstanding this duty to the athlete, the professionally employed team physician also has a duty to her employer. This duty is especially obvious when the team physician is performing an examination to determine if an athlete should be offered a scholarship or should be drafted.[5] These examinations are not being undertaken for the purposes of benefiting the athlete but for the purposes of benefiting the university of professional sports team. This type of examination is analogous to a preemployment examination performed by a physician for the benefit of a potential employer of the examinee. The issue in both cases is whether there is a traditional doctor-patient relationship. Does the physician have a duty to disclose to the examinee the findings of the examination? Most court cases in this area of the law have found that the physician has a duty to conduct the examination with reasonable care in order to discover dangerous conditions within the scope of the examination and then to take reasonable steps to alert the examinee of any dangerous conditions he actually discovers.[6]

Whereas the preparticipation examination in high school athletics may determine who should be excluded from participation, examinations at the collegiate and professional sports levels have potentially more far-reaching consequences. Determinations made by team physicians may have long-term effects on the athlete's ability to qualify for a scholarship, to be drafted by a professional team, and to accumulate future earnings. If a team physician negligently misdiagnoses a condition as more serious than it actually is and the player's career suffers, the team physician may be subject to liability for lost opportunities.[5,7] Therefore, the potential liability present in performing the preparticipation examination on the amateur athlete is increased when performing the examination on collegiate and professional athletes.

The Independence of the Professional or Collegiate Team Physician

Players often challenge the independence of team physicians from team management.[7] The collegiate and the professional team physician may face pressures from coaches, other players, the administration, the owners, and the medical staff (i.e., specialists who benefit from referral patients), all potential beneficiaries of the team physician's services.[8] These pressures may be similar to the pressures felt by volunteer team physicians, but the added pressure of trying to satisfy a employer makes them more intense. The team physician's allegiance must always ultimately be to the best interest of the athlete. Although it is the team physician's job to minimize the time athletes have to stay out of action, team physicians have a greater obligation to keep athletes alive and free from injury.[9] If the well-being of an athlete is in conflict with an interest of a third party, the well-being of the athlete is always paramount.[5] Potential conflicts can be minimized by making it clear from the start that the team physician has the final say regarding any player's participation. It also must be made clear to the employer—if necessary demanded of the employer—that respect for the health of the athlete should be the primary concern.[10]

The Motivation of Money

Almost all athletes at all levels are highly motivated. The collegiate and professional athlete may face the additional motivator of money, either present or future dollars. An athlete may prefer to risk health for the sake of participation and success in the game, motivated by machismo, peer pressure, pride, institutional pressures, and also economic considerations.[5] Money can be and is an important consideration. Athletes don't increase their chances for scholarships, future big earnings, or continued bonuses when they're on the sidelines with an injury. Team physicians treating athletes must keep those powerful motivators in mind when determining the extent of an injury and the time needed for recovery. Athletes may be operating under the concept of no pain, no gain. Their motivations help explain what they are looking for in the way of medical treatment.

The Professional Contract

The team physician's duties and responsibilities are often better defined in a contract at the professional level than the amateur level because the responsibilities are the basis for remuneration. Contracts may spell out the events team physicians who are hired and paid by universities and professional teams are required to attend. The most important clauses in the contract with respect to the professional team physician's ultimate liability concern her ability to exercise independent judgment. The professional team physician's contract should specifically and clearly spell out that the team physician is free to exercise her independent judgment regarding the medical treatment and evaluation of athletes, and this judgment is final and determinative.[5] Other contractual issues are spelled out in chapter 1.

Confidentiality

The issue of confidentiality often arises in professional and collegiate sports. The athlete and the team physician have a confidential physician-patient relationship. But when a team physician is paid by management, a different relationship may exist between the doctor and the athlete. The team physician has two masters to serve: the athlete-patient and the university or professional team management.

As noted in chapter 1, the American Medical Association, through its Judicial Council, admonishes physicians not to reveal confidences entrusted to them unless required to do so by law or, if necessary, to protect the welfare of the individual or the community.[11] In the case of the professional or collegiate team physician, however, because of the scholarships or salaries received by the athletes, the university management or professional team management may have access to their records. This access to the information contained in individual medical records is deemed appropriate. Therefore, discussing the condition of the athlete with management would also probably be viewed as appropriate.[2] However, to ensure that the athlete understands that such information can and will be communicated to the university or professional team management, the team physician may want athletes to sign a release at the beginning of the season, stating that they understand that information about their status that could impact their ability to participate may be communicated to the management. This release may not be legally necessary, but it will go a long way in allowing the team physician some degree of comfort when she communicates information about an athlete to others.

Collegiate and professional team physicians should be careful about giving information to the press. Some professional athletes may be deemed to be public figures and therefore lose some of their right to privacy,[12] but in general, team physicians owe athletes confidentiality. The team physician's paramount obligation must be to the patient, and information disclosed to the press can be potentially financially damaging to the athlete. If the information is erroneous, then the athlete may have a cause of action against the team physician who supplied it.

Chuy v. Philadelphia Eagles Football Club, which was mentioned earlier, is an example of this. Chuy was erroneously diagnosed with Polycythemia Vera and the team physician gave this diagnosis to the press. The court held that there was sufficient evidence to support the jury's determination that the team physician had intentionally or recklessly inflicted mental distress on the plaintiff.

Because of cases like *Chuy*, collegiate and professional teams and team physicians may require athletes to execute a publicity waiver form. Such a form will provide a measure of protection to team physicians who may be

MEMO TO: All Student-Athletes
FROM: Mr. Friendly, Director of Athletic Services
SUBJECT: Release of Personal and Medical Information, and
                    Acknowledgment of Physical Examinations and
                    Athletic Department Policies

It is important to read this carefully before signing. If you have questions, I will be glad to discuss them.

As most of you are aware, current laws protect your right to privacy and your right to be made adequately aware of policies and procedures. The following statements outline the policies of the Athletic Department regarding the gathering and release of information, physical examination procedure, and your acknowledgment you have received a copy of the "Statement of Policy Governing Intercollegiate Athletics" and realize the importance of reading and understanding this document.

   I.   I give my authorization to the registrar, the dean of my college, and my course instructors to release my official transcript and academic records to the Athletic Department with the understanding the Athletic Department will release this information only in cases of academic awards and/or in responding to NCAA or conference requests.

  II.   I authorize the information contained in the Sports Information Office questionnaire to be used by the Athletic Department for press releases, press guide brochures, and official programs. I further permit this information to be released to members of the media.

 III.   I do____do not____give my consent for the team physician, athletic trainers, or other medical personnel of the University to release such information regarding my medical history, record of injury or surgery, record of serious illness, and rehabilitation results as may be requested by the scout or representative of any professional or amateur athletic organization or business organization seeking such information.

 IV.   I understand the Athletic Department has adopted the NCAA policy regarding medical examinations which indicates a full medical examination should be required only under the student-athlete's initial entrance into an institution's intercollegiate program and provided there is a continuous awareness

(continued)

Figure 11.1   A publicity waiver form.

of the health status of the athlete the traditional annual physical examination is not deemed necessary. I further understand if I encounter any medical or orthopedic problems that would exempt me from competing in any Athletic Department sponsored sport I will contact the athletic training staff immediately.

V. By signing this form I acknowledge I have been given a copy of the "Statement of Policy Governing Intercollegiate Athletics" at the University and realize the importance of reading and understanding this document.

| Student's Name (Signature) | Social Security Number | Sport | Date |

Figure 11.1

asked to release or furnish information about athletes under their care. Figure 11.1 contains a publicity waiver form.

Practical Considerations

The most important concept for the collegiate or professional team physician to remember is that the athlete's well-being always comes first, despite intense pressure from the coaches, management, the press, and even the motivated athlete herself to hurry a rehabilitation or return the athlete to participation earlier than otherwise would be considered. If the team physician gives in to those pressures, she is not meeting the duty owed to the athlete, which is to provide for his health and safety first.

Professional team physicians, because they receive compensation for their services, are typically not protected from liability for allegedly negligent acts by Good Samaritan statutes. Professional team physicians may, however, be partially protected from lawsuits by the workers' compensation statutes in their states.

Team physicians who are paid, whether collegiate or professional team physicians, are typically involved with athletes at a higher skill level than team physicians who work with athletes at the amateur level. If the team physician acts in a negligent manner toward these athletes and it results in possible loss of contract or scholarship or negatively impacts future earnings, the team physician may ultimately be found liable for those damages. Team physicians who work with professional athletes or collegiate athletes thus may have liability over and above the liability for negligent acts that result in an injury to a player.

If the press pressures the team physician for information, he should check with the athlete first for permission to relate information to the press.

References

1. Cramer v. Hoffman, 390 F. 2d 19 (2nd Cir. 1968).
2. Berry, R., & Wong, G. (1986). Application of legal principles to persons involved in sports. In *Law and the Business of the Sports Industries: Common Issues in Amateur and Professional Sports*, 2nd ed. 303. Westport, CT: Greenwood Press, Inc.
3. Chuy v. Philadelphia Eagles Football Club, 431 F.Supp. 254 (E.D. Pa. 1977), 595 F. 2d 1265 (1979).
4. Ellis v. Rocky Mountain Empire Sports, Inc., 602 P.2d. 895 (Colo. App. 1979).
5. King, J., (1981). The duty and the standard of care for team physicians. *Houston Law Review*, **18**, 657-705.
6. Russell, C. (1987). Legal and ethical conflicts arising from the team physician's dual obligations to the athlete and management. *Seton Hall Legislative Journal*, **10**(2).
7. Davis, J. (1992). "Fixing" the standard of care: Motivated athletes and medical malpractice. *American Journal of Trial Advocacy*, **12**, 215.
8. Kass, R. (1980). Ethical dilemmas in the care of the ill. *Journal of the American Medical Association*, **244**, 1811-1813.
9. Fairbanks (1979, August). Return to sports participation. *Physician and Sports Medicine*, 71-82.
10. Olgilvie (1977, April). Walking the perilous path of the team psychologist. *Physician and Sports Medicine*, **5**(1), 62-66.
11. American Medical Association. (1969, updated 1992). *Opinions and reports of the Judicial Council* (p. 56). Chicago: Author.
12. Morley, M. B. (1982). Malpractice on the sidelines. *Journal of Communications and Entertainment Law*, 579-600.

CHAPTER 12

Risk Management

A physician, volunteering as a team physician for a local high school, saw a football receiver in his office who had sustained a mild rotator cuff tear. The physician appropriately diagnosed it and called a colleague, an orthopedic surgeon, for advice. She told him the athlete should use a shoulder harness for the remainder of the season to protect his healing shoulder. The team physician was unfamiliar with the application of the harness and simply instructed his nurse to "give the boy the harness that is coming over from Dr. Smith's office." Because the athlete was not a regular patient, the physician did not have a chart made up and made no record of his treatment of the athlete.

The athlete applied the harness incorrectly when he went out for practice the next day and severely reinjured his shoulder, necessitating surgery.

Questions:

▮ Is the team physician liable for his failure to appropriately communicate with the athlete?

▮ What will the team physician use in the courtroom to defend himself, having failed to chart anything related to his evaluation and treatment?

▮ What are the appropriate records for a team physician to keep?

As in any other area of medical practice, risk management is the key to preventing lawsuits in sports medicine. Technically, *risk management* is an insurance term used to describe various measures to resolve, reduce, or transfer risks that predictably occur in any particular underwriting line. It is a retrospective identification of monetary loss based on past occurrences among the insured.[1] In reality, risk management is nothing more or less than competent care of patients and documentation of it. By managing the risk of lawsuits, team physicians can minimize their exposure to potential liability.

Risk management in sports medicine is a process of accomplishing two separate but interrelated tasks:

1. Recognizing the primary risks associated with any given activity and taking all reasonable steps to eliminate or reduce them
2. Recognizing that, despite a best effort, not all injuries can be avoided and, therefore, taking appropriate steps to maximize the likelihood of successfully defending whatever lawsuits may arise[2]

Four key elements of good risk management are

- compassion,
- communication,
- competence, and
- charting.[3]

Each of these elements is essential to good risk management; however, compassion and communication are especially important because studies show that 70% of the reasons patients sue are because of communication and attitude problems with their treating physicians.[4]

Compassion

Physicians who have good relationships with their patients are less likely to be sued than physicians who have poor relationships. Physicians who demonstrate a deep concern for their patients are often able to avoid litigation, even when a poor outcome occurs. The one element necessary for every lawsuit is a dissatisfied patient. Patients find it difficult to sue a physician they like and one they believe cares about them.[3] Developing rapport with patients, whether they are athletes or nonathletes, enhances the physician-patient relationship. Rudeness and arrogance not only prevent rapport, they also may cause the athlete to be especially angry when something goes wrong. When a bad result occurs or something unexpected happens, athletes may consider filing a lawsuit just to get back at the physician for his attitude, yet the same athlete may have accepted an error of medical judgment from a more caring physician. Human nature historically punishes arrogance and forgives humility.[5]

Communication

Informed consent, a method of communication, is the cornerstone of good communication with patients and touches on all aspects of patient care.

Team physicians must educate athletes and, when appropriate, their parents or guardians about the options of treatment, likely outcomes, and significant risks of each option.[3]

This education is the hallmark of informed consent. In athletics, many parents and players expect the risks of participation to be lower than what they really are. Effective communication with athletes and parents can help to ensure that they are completely informed about the most common risks inherent in certain sports. If an athlete demands to be allowed to participate in a sport against the recommendation of the team physician, informing her of the risks of participation is absolutely essential. If an athlete or his guardian elects to participate even in the face of the team physician's recommendations otherwise, the physician should ask the athlete or his guardian to execute an exculpatory waiver or risk release if appropriate in that state.

One of the areas of risk for team physicians that relates to communication is in the use of consultants. If time is important, and it almost always is in athletics, the team physician should consider calling the consultant to assure a prompt visit. Then the team physician should clearly communicate the consultant's role to the athlete. The team physician defines the scope of the consultation. The consultation is just that, a consultation, and the team physician is ultimately responsible for determining what treatment or participation options the athlete will pursue. If the team physician disagrees with the consultant's advice, she should document the disagreement and its basis.[6]

Competence

Some physicians who are sued for medical malpractice are sued because, for a variety of reasons, they did commit malpractice.[3] Perhaps the physician, with the best intentions, administered inappropriate care. If the minimally competent physician in the same specialty in similar circumstances would not have done the same thing, then the well-intentioned physician may well have committed a negligent act. A physician who commits a negligent act, as discussed in chapters 1 and 2, may be liable for malpractice.

One of the best means for team physicians to avoid liability for malpractice is to maintain clinical competence in the field. Sports medicine is no different than any other type of medicine. All areas of medicine are constantly in flux, with new methodologies for diagnosis, treatment, and rehabilitation being developed continuously. New practice guidelines are being developed constantly. All new developments in sports medicine and other related areas of medicine impact on the team physician. The public, and ultimately the court, expects the team physician to maintain clinical competence and to practice in reasonable conformity with new developments in the field. Team physicians must make every effort to maintain clinical competence by attending workshops and keeping up with the literature in the field of sports medicine.

Charting

The medical record is the physician's biggest ally in court.[3] According to one estimate, 35% to 40% of all medical malpractice suits are rendered indefensible by problems with the medical record. A bad result added to a bad record equals liability, regardless of the facts and the standard of care practiced.[7] Medical records take on added significance because lawsuits take anywhere from 2 to 10 years after the incident in question to come to trial.[8] This may be long after a team physician has any recall of the events in question. A case filed in Hawaii in 1985 alleged medical malpractice by a surgeon during a 1962 procedure![9]

Effective record keeping serves two purposes. It enables the team physician, the trainer, and (in some cases) other school personnel to understand and follow what is occurring with an athlete—a medical purpose. As the team physician's biggest ally, it provides written evidence of what occurred with an athlete—a legal purpose.[3] The development and implementation of comprehensive record-keeping systems will enhance the effectiveness of organizational communication while helping to minimize the threat of a lawsuit arising from the failure to adequately document the nature and extent of care provided to an injured athlete.[10]

Some general points about record keeping should be remembered. Physicians should write legibly. This seems to go without saying, but many physicians continue to make illegible entries into charts. Picture the following scenario: A physician is on the stand at his own trial and the plaintiff's attorney asks the physician to read an entry he made on the patient's chart. The defendant physician, squirming on the stand, cannot even read his own writing. The inability to read his own illegible chart can markedly diminish a physician's credibility with a jury. The jury may view the physician as "sloppy," and if the physician is sloppy in record keeping, maybe he is also sloppy in other areas. See page 163 for more on the importance of record keeping.

Medical records can win or lose a lawsuit. They are the single most important piece of evidence in any medical malpractice trial. Careless record keeping may sink a good physician, and meticulous record keeping may persuade a jury to favor a physician they otherwise have thought made a mistake.[11]

Common Problems with Medical Records

Even if the physician does keep a medical record for an athlete, some common problems can markedly reduce the record's value in defending a medical malpractice case.

Altering the Record

One of the first things a physician does when receiving information indicating that a lawsuit is likely is to review the chart.[12] This chart review may tempt the physician to make corrections or addendums. Under no circumstances should charts be altered once they are in dispute. There is no way to credibly defend an altered chart. Altering a patient's medical record to explain or justify a diagnosis or treatment, even if done in good faith, can create a presumption of fraud and attack a physician's credibility in the eyes of a jury.[11]

In a case regarding the appropriate or inappropriate administration of penicillin to a child who subsequently developed fatal anaphylaxis, the defendant physicians made an addendum to the record in a different-colored pen, which almost beckoned the plaintiff's attorney to notice the change![13] Plaintiffs' attorneys have been known to date the ink used to prove that an entry was made after the original entry. In case after case involving altered medical records, physicians have lost malpractice suits because they altered the record although their case management seemed to be appropriate. Never alter a medical record.

Team Physician Medical Records

Team physicians' medical record keeping for athletes cared for in their offices should not differ from record keeping for other patients in the office. In other words, it should be as involved and as detailed as possible. However, often team physicians render care on the sidelines or in the locker room. Just because the site of the rendered care is atypical, the team physician still has a duty to document the care rendered. In an emergent situation or where immediate note taking or dictating is not feasible, the team physician should execute complete notes regarding the treatment or situation as soon as possible. At a minimum, the records should note the athlete's name, sport, nature of the injury or illness, date, immediate treatment, and treatment and rehabilitation recommended.[14]

Pertinent original medical records should be kept at the physician's office. Where applicable, copies of progress notes or test results may be kept in the training room. Access to these records should be limited to appropriate individuals such as the trainer and possibly student trainers.

Informed consent documents, assumption of risk documents, and exculpatory waivers should be included in the athlete's record and kept at the team physician's office. Copies of these may be kept at the school, college, or stadium.

The underlying reason for effective record keeping is good communication. This good communication includes not only communication between the team physician and the athlete but also between the team physician, the trainers, the parents, and the coaching staff. One of the most common allegations against medical practitioners is lack of effective communication, which often has its basis in a lack of effective record keeping.[14]

Record Retention

One of the most important reasons for retaining patient records is for self-defense.[15] How long to retain medical records is a difficult question to answer in the practice of any type of medicine, and sports medicine is no exception. Unfortunately, the answer depends on the statute of limitations, which varies from state to state. The statute of limitations sets specific periods of time within which lawsuits must be instigated.[8] The statute of limitations usually is triggered by either the incident that gives rise to a claim of negligence or by when an error should have been detected by the patient. For instance, the amputation of the wrong limb is a triggering incident and is immediately notable by a patient. A sponge left in a surgical patient may be undetected by the patient for years until it begins to cause complications. The statute of limitations generally ranges from 2 to 3 years in most states; however, this general guideline is modified in certain key instances, the most important of which is minority. Some states allow an injured child to sue up to 3 years after reaching the age of majority, which may be when the child is 22. Hence when the athlete is a minor a cause of action may remain valid for years after it occurred.[16]

The best way to ensure that records are retained long enough is to keep them permanently, but this may not be practical. Team physicians should consult with attorneys in their state who are familiar with the statute of limitations before deciding to obliterate or otherwise destroy records.

Practical Considerations

The four C's of risk management, compassion, communication, competence, and charting, so helpful for all physicians in all areas of medicine, also help the team physician avoid lawsuits. Of course, there are no guarantees that a physician who practices flawless medicine, communicates well with patients and medical personnel, and keeps stellar records will not be sued. However, the likelihood of a successful lawsuit against such a physician is very low.

Risk management has many definitions. It really isn't what plaintiffs' lawyers claim—the practice of "defensive" medicine. Risk management is simply the practice of competent clinical medicine and documentation of the same.

It is a tenet of good medicine that the physicians communicate effectively with their patients. Informed consent is part of medicine, and good medical practice demands full and adequate informed consent communication.

The public has a right to expect physicians to practice competently, and thus physicians have a duty to keep up with the changing developments in sports medicine literature and to attend and participate in the latest workshops about sports medicine care.

Charting is the bane of almost all physicians, and team physicians are not excepted. Charting is tedious, time consuming, and often seems to be wasteful. Yet charts are the team physician's biggest ally in court. Three rules of record keeping apply to all medical practitioners: If it is not in the record, it did not happen; if the record is illegible, it is worthless; and if the record is unorganized, it is worthless.

Team physicians would do well to carry a dictaphone or a note pad while on the sidelines or at practice to note athletes evaluated and treatment or advice rendered at the scene. The physician can fill in more detail later, but making meaningful notes at the time of an occurrence will be invaluable to ensuring that the record is adequate.

The Importance of Record Keeping

Some general principles related to record keeping bear repeating here.

Write legibly. This seems to go without saying, but many physicians continue to make illegible entries into charts. A considerable portion of most handwritten records are illegible, and up to 80% of all physicians' signatures are illegible. The consequences of illegible handwriting may be potentially catastrophic if a patient receives less than optimal management because of an illegible entry. It also may be catastrophic if a record fails to back up a premise of the physician's defense because it is illegible.

Use only widely recognized abbreviations. If an abbreviation is to be used repeatedly during an entry, it should be written out completely the first time it is used.

Use SOAP formats. S is for subjective complaints; O is for objective findings; A is for assessment; and P is for plan of treatment. SOAP notes are now the widely accepted appropriate format for progress notes no matter what the physician's specialty.

Use objective language. It does not look very good if a defendant physician on the witness stand has to read disparaging comments about the defendant that may have been written in the chart.

Include the date and time of the progress notes and sign them. A dated and timed progress note can corroborate testimony.

Document any procedures recommended and the patient's response to the recommendation. If the patient refuses the recommended procedure, note both the refusal and the fact that the risks of refusal were discussed.

Note noncompliance by patients and efforts at seeking compliance.

Include recommendations for follow-up care. This includes recommendations for physical therapy, consultations and return office visits.

Proofread dictated medical records. Writing "dictated but not read" on the record or claiming that the chart was not read does not provide any protection in court. Make appropriate corrections and fill in blanks.

Note recommendations by consultants that you disagree with along with the rationale for the disagreement.

Include telephone calls in the chart.

References

1. Gibbs, R.F. (1989, September). Ambulatory care risk management. *Medical Malpractice Prevention*, pp. 14-16.
2. Dougherty, N. (1989). Risk management in sports medicine programs. *The Sports Medicine Standards and Malpractice Reporter*, 1(3), 47-55.
3. American Academy of Family Physicians Committee on Professional Liability. (1986). *Family physicians and obstetrical malpractice* (p. 1). Kansas City, MO: Author.
4. American Academy of Family Physicians Committee on Professional Liability. (Not yet released). *Risk management and the family physician* (2nd ed.) (p. 2). Kansas City, MO: Author.
5. Tennenhouse, D., & Kasher, M. (1989). *Risk prevention skills* (p. 83). Florida: Tennenhouse Professional Publications.
6. Consultants and the risk of malpractice. (1991, March). *Ohio Medicine*, 87, 141-142.

7. Good records can be strongest malpractice defense. (1983, January). *Michigan Medicine*, 6-8.

8. American Medical Association. (1990). *Grand rounds on medical malpractice* (pp. 50-51). Chicago: Author.

9. Napier, P., & Napier, B. (1989, January). Medical charts and malpractice: How to avoid costly errors and omissions. *Hawaii Medical Journal*, **48**(1).

10. Hawkins, J. (1989). Sports medicine record keeping: The key to effective communication and documentation. *Sports Medicine Standards and Malpractice Reporter*, **1**(2), 31-35.

11. Barton, H. (1990, May). Medical records can win or lose a malpractice case. *Texas Medicine*, **86**(5).

12. Danner, D. (1986). *A primer for physicians* (p. 4). Rochester, NY: The Lawyers Cooperative Publishing Co.

13. Rotan v. Greenbaum, 273 F. 2d 830 (D.C., 1959).

14. Hawkins, J.D. (1989). Sports medicine recordkeeping: The key to effective documentation. *Sports Medicine Standards and Malpractice Reporter*, **1**(2), 31-35.

15. Berg, R. (1990, April 6). Are you awash in medical records? *American Medical News*, p. 9.

16. *Protective pointers, keeping the physician out of court* (p. 18). Fort Wayne, IN: The Medical Protective Company.

Checklist for the Team Physician

Prior to the School Year

✓ Has the team physician met the coaches and the athletic director prior to assuming the responsibilities of team physician?

✓ Has the team physician conducted or participated in a meeting with the athletes and their parents prior to the beginning of the season, fully discussing the risks of participation, the responsibilities of the athletes, and the responsibilities of the team physician?

✓ Has a contract been executed with the school or college outlining the responsibilities of and remuneration or lack of remuneration for the team physician?

✓ Has the team physician offered to participate in the evaluation and choice of protective equipment for the team?

The Preparticipation Physical

✓ Has the team physician ascertained that the history of the athlete is fully documented in the preparticipation history form?

✓ Does the physical examination include a musculoskeletal examination and is the examination conducted in a quiet environment?

✓ Are the results of the examination fully disclosed to the athlete and to parents if the athlete is underage?

✓ Are appropriate recommendations communicated to the coaches and trainers?

At the Game Site

✓ Have appropriately trained personnel been identified to assist in the provision of on-site emergency medical care?

✓ Has adequate on-site emergency equipment been provided?

✓ Is adequate emergency transportation with appropriately trained personnel available on-site or on call?

✓ Are appropriate communication mechanisms available to summon emergency transportation?

✓ Have appropriate hospital facilities with well-trained personnel been identified?

✓ Have appropriate consultative services been identified?

Risk Management

✓ Communication
Is the communication plan well defined and do all the trainers and other medical personnel understand their responsibilities with respect to communications?

✓ Documentation
Is there a method to document treatment given to athletes from opposing teams? Is there a method to document the treatment rendered and advice given to athletes in the locker room?

Ascertaining State Law

✓ Are the state law requirements for informed consent known?

✓ Is it known how the state views exculpatory waivers, especially those executed by athletes?

✓ Does the state have a specific Good Samaritan statute that applies to team physicians? If so, does it also apply to preparticipation physical examinations?

INDEX

Parenthetical page references following page references to end notes indicate pages where the case or law referred to in an end note is discussed, but not named.

ABOUT THE AUTHOR

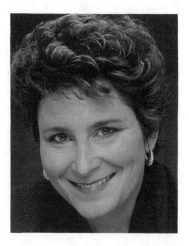

Elizabeth M. Gallup is a board certified family physician and a licensed attorney in two states. She is also a former high school and college team physician. In 1989, she joined the American Academy of Family Physicians and served as its Assistant General Counsel. During the three years she was with the Academy, Dr. Gallup developed a department of state legislation, directed the department of professional liability, and participated in the American Medical Association Medical Specialty Society Professional Liability project.

After leaving the Academy, Dr. Gallup became the medical director of Trans World Airlines, a position she held until 1993 when she joined William M. Mercer, Inc., as a health care consultant. In 1994, Dr. Gallup was appointed senior vice president for physician and business development at Shawnee Mission Medical Center. She is also the CEO of the medical center's physician hospital organization.

Dr. Gallup is one of the founding members of the American Medical Society for Sports Medicine. She continues to practice medicine as the medical director for the Kansas City (Missouri) Free Health Clinic. She is also an associate clinical professor of family medicine at the University of Missouri at Kansas City. Dr. Gallup earned her medical degree from The Ohio State University in 1981 and her law degree from the University of Toledo in 1986. Her favorite leisure-time activities include exercising, reading, and writing.